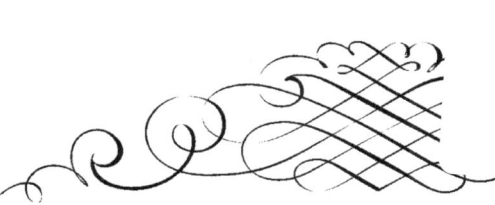
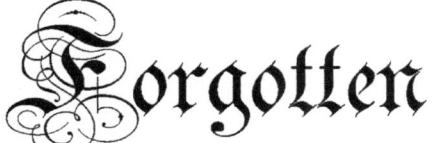 

ISBN 978-1-333-08144-7
PIBN 10128553

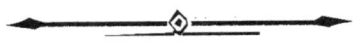

English
Français
Deutsche
Italiano
Español
Português

www.forgottenbooks.com

Mythology Photography **Fiction**
Fishing Christianity **Art** Cooking
Essays Buddhism Freemasonry
Medicine **Biology** Music **Ancient
Egypt** Evolution Carpentry Physics
Dance Geology **Mathematics** Fitness
Shakespeare **Folklore** Yoga Marketing
Confidence Immortality Biographies
Poetry **Psychology** Witchcraft
Electronics Chemistry History **Law**
Accounting **Philosophy** Anthropology
Alchemy Drama Quantum Mechanics
Atheism Sexual Health **Ancient History**
Entrepreneurship Languages Sport
Paleontology Needlework Islam
Metaphysics Investment Archaeology
Parenting Statistics Criminology
Motivational

DISEASES

OF THE

Lungs, Bronchi and Pleura

BY

H. WORTHINGTON PAIGE, M. D.

LECTURER ON THEORY AND PRACTICE OP MEDICINE IN THE NEW YORK HOMŒO-
PATHIC MEDICAL COLLEGE AND HOSPITAL; MEMBER OF THE ATTENDING
STAFF TO THE FLOWER HOSPITAL, THE HAHNEMANN HOSPITAL,
AND THE LAURA FRANKLIN FREE HOSPITAL FOR CHILDREN;
LATE ASSISTANT SURGEON TO THE THROAT
DEPARTMENT OP THE NEW YORK
OPHTHALMIC HOSPITAL.

PHILADELPHIA.
BOERICKE & TAFEL.
1904.

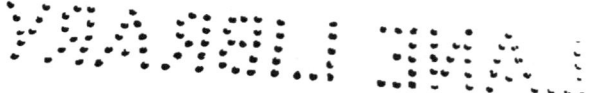

To

JAMES MONTFORT SCHLEY, M. D.,

THIS LITTLE VOLUME IS DEDICATED BY THE

AUTHOR IN GRATEFUL APPRECIATION

OF HIS FRIENDSHIP AND IN MODEST

RECOGNITION OF HIS STERLING

SERVICES TO HUMANITY

AND THE MEDICAL

PROFESSION.

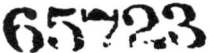

PREFACE.

This small volume is designed to be a concise text-book embodying the essential facts relating to the subjects treated. These are told in a practical way and arranged in a convenient form in the hope that it may prove a useful handbook for the busy practitioner or student. Unproven theories are not discussed. Well established facts only are given, and these without unprofitable elaboration. The methods described under general treatment are the most approved, and the formulæ given have been used and found efficacious. It would be impossible in a volume of this size to give all the remedies that might be indicated in any given condition, so the author has limited himself to mentioning those most frequently useful. Standard writings have been consulted in the preparation of this book, with the endeavor to make it represent the essence of current opinion. Hoping that it may find a place among the physician's useful reference books, it is entrusted to the kindly criticism of the profession.

H. WORTHINGTON PAIGE.

New York City, November, 1904.

CONTENTS.

SECTION III.

DISEASES OF THE LUNGS.

SECTION IV.

DISEASES OF THE PLEURA.

SECTION V.

DISEASES OF THE MEDIASTINUM.

I.

Diseases of the Trachea.

DISEASES OF THE TRACHEA.

TRACHEITIS.

Definition.—Tracheitis is a catarrhal inflammation of the mucous membrane lining the trachea. It may be acute or chronic and is usually associated with a similar inflammation in the larynx or bronchi, but may exist independently.

Etiology.—It is caused by the same influences—exposure with lack of resistance or the inhalation of irritating matter—that would excite a laryngitis or bronchitis, or may occur secondarily by extension of either of the latter.

Pathology.—Tracheitis passes through the usual phases common to catarrhal inflammations elsewhere. A first stage of dry congested and swollen mucosa and the second stage of relaxation, free mucous or muco-purulent secretion, with which the inflammation subsides.

Physical Signs.—Auscultation reveals a greatly increased harshness, roughness and strident quality to the tracheal breathing. Later there are coarse rattling rales.

Diagnosis.—Interference with vocalization, hoarseness or aphonia supplemented by a laryngoscopic examination will reveal whether the larynx is involved or not and auscultation will show if there be associated bronchitis. The constitutional disturbance is more pronounced in the latter.

Symptoms.— In the early stage, chilliness, fever, shifting pains, thirst and headache. The tracheal cough is characteristic—deep, hollow, tubular and rough, sounding as if something was being torn out, but not as painful as it sounds. There may be tracheal soreness and sensitiveness to touch or inhalation of cold air. In the later stage secretion is abundant as a rule and easily expectorated. The so-called "death rattle" so often heard just before death in a variety of conditions is merely an excess of secretion in the trachea, due to relaxation of the mucosa, and which the patient is too weak to expectorate. The "tickling in the throat pit" and "tickling behind the sternum," so often quoted as causing cough, does not necessarily indicate tracheitis, but is usually a nervous reflex symptom, exciting a bronchial rather than a tracheal cough.

General Treatment.—The management of tracheitis should be the same as of acute bronchitis. There are several remedies, however, especially indicated.

Remedies.— *Bryonia.*—Dry, hard cough of rough tearing quality. Scanty expectoration, but much tracheal soreness, rawness and pain. The cough causes bursting frontal headache. The first remedy to be thought of in the early stage.

Drosera.—Deep, hoarse cough, rather paroxysmal, with muco-purulent expectoration and rough, scraped sensation in the trachea.

Hepar sulphur.—Dry, rough, hoarse cough with audible wheezing. The dry stage is merging into the looser condition. Patient very sensitive to cold.

Iodine.—Hollow, croupy cough with rawness and pain in the trachea and wheezing, difficult respiration. Scrofulous, catarrhal subjects.

Kali bichromicum.—Hoarse cough with coarse, rattling tracheal rales and the expectoration, with much effort, of quantities of tenacious, yellow mucus. Late stages. Weak, phlegmatic, hepatic people.

Spongia.—Early stages. Great dryness. Hoarseness or aphonia with constriction. Dry, barking, croupy cough. Respiration short and labored, especially inspiration; nightly aggravation.

STENOSIS OF THE TRACHEA.

Definition.— Tracheal stenosis is a contraction of the trachea from changes in its own walls or the pressure of diseased conditions in neighboring structures.

Etiology.—The most usual causes are goitre, enlarged lymphatic glands, aneurism of the arch of the aorta, tumors, abscesses, or cancer in the mediastinum, or cancer of the lung.

Symptoms.—The cardinal symptom of tracheal stenosis is dyspnœa of an inspiratory character. All the accessory respiratory muscles may be brought into play during inspiration, while expiration is smooth and unobstructed. There is a peculiar whistling, crowing note produced during inspiration and the vibration of the column of air imparts a distinct thrill to the trachea. The vesicular sounds are diminished and masked by the tracheal sounds. The voice is weak and muffled, because the air is interrupted and lessened in force while passing the vocal chords.   The laryngoscope is the best aid to diagnosis, in locating and determining the cause. Respiratory distress gradually increases with the increase of the underlying cause of obstruction.   There may be periods of acute exacerbation also, with alarming symptoms. The usual symptoms of dyspnœa are present, *i. e.*, face anxious, pale and covered with sweat, or cyanotic, with movement of the alæ nasi, the pulse rapid and weak, all those well known symptoms indicating distress for need of air.   The course, duration and ultimate outcome depend upon the nature and progress of the causative factor.

Treatment.—This depends wholly upon the cause of the stenosis.

II.

Diseases of the Bronchi.

II.

DISEASES OF THE BRONCHI.

ACUTE BRONCHITIS.

Definition.—Acute bronchitis is an acute catarrhal inflammation of the mucous membrane lining the larger and medium sized bronchial tubes, usually involving the trachea to a greater or less extent (tracheitis). It is a very common disorder, and while not serious in the healthy adult, becomes of grave import in infancy and old age, owing to the tendency to extension, with resulting pulmonary complications. When attacking the finer tubes its manifestations become more severe and will be described separately (see Capillary Bronchitis). It is bilateral and may occur as an independent affection, or as a complication in association with other diseases.

Etiology.—Acute bronchitis is a common result of "catching cold" and is most frequently the downward extension of an acute coryza. It is most prevalent in the changeable weather of early spring and autumn. Like all catarrhal affections, it is prone to attack delicate people, victims of malnutrition, those who live in unhygienic surroundings and especially persons exhibiting a strumous diathesis. Some, otherwise healthy subjects, seem peculiarly susceptible and develop acute bronchitis upon the slightest exposure. Among the exciting causes are: wetting the feet, chilling the body after warm bathing, going out from a warm room when perspiring, exposure after singing or prolonged speaking, the draughts in cars, insufficient clothing, etc. A sedentary life, enervating habits, bad drainage, or improper food are all potent factors in lessening the power to resist. *Too* much clothing, a fondness for warm baths, super-heated homes and especially close confinement therein during the winter months render people particularly susceptible to the changeable spring weather. Hot-house kept children by over-zealous parents fall easy victims. The extremes of life, with their lesser power to resist, furnish the larger quota of cases of bronchitis. The inhalation of irritating foreign material, common dust or that of steel or coal, pollen, cotton, etc., or, again, irritating gases, chlorine, ammonia, illuminating gas, not infrequently excites a simple bronchitis. It often occurs also in association with other diseases; notably, measles, whooping cough, typhoid fever and variola. The bronchitis of asthma, heart disease, chronic nephritis, gout and various nervous diseases, is of the chronic type.

Pathology.—The initial lesion is a hyperæmia of the mucous membrane, varying in degree according to the severity of the attack. In mild cases there may be only limited areas of arborescent redness, but in the severe cases the mucous membrane becomes turgescent, smooth, shiny and swollen, with œdema of the submucosa. During the initial hyperæmia there is dryness of the surface, followed in a few hours by the exudation of clear, transparent mucus. As the disease progresses the secretion becomes richer in mucin and exfoliated ciliated epithelia, hence thicker and more tenacious, gradually changing to muco-purulent character, yellowish in color from the presence of pus cells. If of greenish tint it is due to blood coloring matter, though blood rarely appears in acute bronchitis except as it stains or streaks the mucus, *i. e.*, in minute quantities.

Symptoms. — Acute bronchitis begins with the familiar symptoms of general cold, headache, coryza, sore throat, hoarseness, general pains and aching, chilliness, accompanied by slight fever. The temperature rarely rises above 101° to 102° in a simple bronchitis, but the amount of cough and bronchial irritation is not always in proportion to the fever, some cases with very severe cough showing but little rise of temperature and vice versa. The patient experiences sensations of tightness, oppression, rawness and soreness, amounting in severe attacks to thoracic pain. The diaphragm and abdominal muscles become sore and lame if the cough is severe and all the chest symptoms are aggravated by coughing. The *cough* is a constant symptom. At first it is short, hacking and dry, frequent and distressing, causing pain and soreness of the chest and abdomen and in some cases vomiting and involuntary urination. During this early stage the expectoration is scanty, thin, transparent mucus. Later, the cough softens, becomes gradually looser, the soreness and distressing symptoms diminish and the expectoration changes, becoming freer, more abundant and muco-purulent or purulent in character. The condition terminates favorably in a period varying from a few days to two weeks, with proper care and treatment.

Physical Signs.—In mild cases these may be absent altogether. Percussion yields negative results in simple bronchitis. Palpation gives bronchial fremitus. Auscultation shows in the early stage, rough, accentuated breathing, with dry rales, varying from sibilant to sonorous, according to the size of the tubes involved. With the development of freer secretion, the rales become moist, bubbling or rattling, coarse or fine, according to the size of the tubes affected and changing in character or location upon coughing. Examine the base of both lungs daily and watch the temperature carefully during acute bronchitis in infancy and old age, to discover first evidence of capillary or pulmonary extension.

Complications.—These are not uncommon in acute bronchitis, especially in infants and the aged. The most frequent are capillary extension, broncho-pneumonia, atelectasis, asthma, emphysema and disturbances of circulation.

Diagnosis. — The suddenness of attack, method of onset, the low temperature, the absence of consolidation or severe constitutional symptoms usually make the diagnosis clear. The danger lies in the fact that the ease with which the presence of bronchitis is determined may lead to the overlooking of some more grave coexisting condition. The rales of simple bronchitis are usually bilateral; if unilateral suspicion is felt of some localized lesion, pneumonic or phthisical. Phthisis and broncho-pneumonia are frequently ushered in with the symptoms of acute bronchitis, hence it is well to examine cases of supposed simple bronchitis carefully for evidence of pulmonary consolidation. Percussion dullness does not appear in uncomplicated bronchitis. Extension of the disease to the smaller bronchioles or pulmonary vesicles is marked by rise of temperature and severity of symptoms

—dyspnœa, dusky color to the skin and systemic depression.

Prognosis.—In uncomplicated bronchitis the prognosis is always favorable. It never leads to a fatal termination except in the extremes of life. In gouty subjects or those who are debilitated it has a marked tendency to become chronic. If complications arise by extension to the finer tubes or air vesicles the prognosis is more grave, the complication then becoming the important factor. Pulmonary involvement is particularly apt to occur in alcoholic habitues or during the course of measles or whooping cough.

General Treatment.—"If a patient has a temperature above normal keep him in bed," is a wise axiom, especially in acute troubles. While acute bronchitis usually yields promptly to treatment, the fact that a certain proportion of cases prove obstinate and protracted and not infrequently lead into more serious conditions emphasizes the importance of giving the most simple cases careful attention. Warmth, rest in bed and an even temperature, all favor early subsidence of the inflammation and freer secretion. In cases marked by soreness or pain, a mustard plaster or flaxseed poulticing is most excellent. During the early stage, with soreness, oppression and racking cough, moist air gives great relief. Inhalation of the steam arising from, ℞. Menthol, grs. x; Tr. Benzoin, ʒi; Aqua, ℥xvi, in a croup-kettle, teapot or open vessel is of much benefit.

If the cough is dry, incessant, painful and fatiguing, robbing the patient of rest and sleep, especially in debilitated subjects, a palliative will give happy results and favor prompt recovery. The following is reliable and satisfactory: ℞. Codeia, grs. iii to iv; Syr. Yerba Santa, ℥iv. S. One teaspoonful every three or four hours as required.

Heroin Muriate in $\frac{1}{12}$ to $\frac{1}{24}$ grain doses in tablet or vehicle as above, is very efficacious as a nervous sedative and does not inhibit secretion. In the aged or those who are enfeebled or ill nourished, a severe cough may prove exhausting, in which case quiet is imperative and concentrated liquid nourishment at regular intervals with stimulation should be employed.

Remedies.—*Aconite.*—Early stage, alternating fever and chilliness; thirst, restlessness and anxiety; shooting pains here and there; short, dry, tickling cough; constant laryngeal irritation.

Belladonna.—Dry, tearing, spasmodic cough; worse at night; waking from sleep and keeping awake, in children followed by crying. Face flushes and eyes suffuse during cough, with throbbing headache. Involuntary micturition during cough.

Antimonium iodide.—Excellent remedy in simple bronchitis with profuse muco-purulent expectoration. Less oppression than *Ant. tart.*, because expectoration is easier.

Antimonium tartaricum.—Similar in action to *Ipecac*, but the condition is more severe. Smaller bronchial tubes affected, being filled with muco-purulent secretion which the patient is unable to raise. Great dyspnœa from suppressed expectoration, cannot get air and has to sit up in bed; oppression temporarily relieved by expectoration. Chest filled with fine, rattling rales. Sweat, weakness and cyanosis. Especially useful in children and the aged.

Bryonia alba.—Inflammation of the trachea and larger bronchi. Hard, dry, tearing cough, causing frontal headache. Chest is tight, painful and sore. Respiration oppressed and cough suppressed, because both cause sharp, sticking pains in chest. Patient lies quiet, as motion, talking or deep breathing causes cough and the chest is too painful. Also excellent for hard morning cough with free expectoration, though cough causes pain and leaves bronchial soreness.

Causticum.—Short, dry, hacking cough, worse toward night, with laryngeal rawness. Involuntary emission of urine when coughing. Hoarseness or loss of voice, particularly in the morning.

Drosera.—Violent paroxysms of coughing following each other in rapid succession. Muco-purulent expectoration. Roughness of voice with hoarseness and cough of a deep bass character.

Ferrum phosphoricum.—Fever, with less thirst, restlessness and irritability than *Aconite*, but more prostration. Chest tight, raw and sore; blood-tinged mucus. Thin, phthisical subjects.

Hepar sulphur.—Hoarse cough (between dry and loose), general wheezing and huskiness throughout the chest. (Not the rattling of *Ipec.* or *Ant. tart.*) Moderate, yellowish expectoration, especially in the morning. Other catarrhal symptoms present with evidence of strumous type; nasal stoppage from hypertrophied turbinateds or adenoids; enlarged tonsils and submaxillary glands. Patient is very sensitive to cold, and removal of covering or other exposure aggravates cough or precipitates the attack.

Ipecac.—One of the best remedies for catarrhal affections of the respiratory tract as inflammation subsides and exudation takes place. Audible, bubbling rales throughout the larger and medium bronchi. Cough spasmodic and paroxysmal, often exciting gagging or vomiting, with free expectoration. In children the cough is suffocative and the patient may become cyanotic during the paroxysm.

Kali bichromicum.—Remedy for the later stages with large amount of tough mucus in the larynx, trachea and larger bronchi. Rough, hoarse voice with stuffy, hoarse cough and expectoration of thick, tenacious, yellow or yellow-green mucus. Prostration, yellow furred tongue and offensive breath. Especially the bronchial catarrh of old people with tenacious expectoration, disgusting gagging effort and offensive odor.

Kali carbonicum.—Hoarseness and cough with the typical tenacious expectoration of the *Kalis*, its particular indication being sticking pains in the chest when coughing and early morning aggravation.

Phosphorus.—Hard, dry, hacking cough from tickling in the throat pit, with scanty expectoration of frothy mucus or mucus tinged with blood. Respiration is short and difficult from tightness and oppression across chest. Larynx is involved with hoarseness or aphonia. Speaking causes a sense of soreness in the larynx and trachea. Cough grows worse toward evening with increase of hoarseness.

Pulsatilla.—Dry night cough relieved by sitting up in bed. Loose cough with expectoration of yellow mucus. Pale, delicate females with chilliness and menstrual irregularities.

Rumex crispus.—Incessant, dry cough, due to irritation in the throat pit, worse in the evening and after lying down. Cough aggravated by pressure, talking and inhaling cold air. There is a sense of rawness and soreness in the larynx and behind the sternum.

Sanguinaria.—Severe hacking cough with pain in the breast and sense of tickling and dryness. Burning and pain in the nose with intense dryness or watery coryza.

Spongia.—Hollow, barking, croupy cough with burning rawness and pain in the larynx and trachea. The hoarseness and croupy character of the voice and cough, showing laryngeal involvement, is the great indication for *Spongia*, especially with the night attack or aggravation.

Sticta and *Hyoscyamus.*—To be thought of for a dry, hacking cough from tickling in the larynx and bronchi. The *Sticta* cough is due to great dryness and hyperæmia of the nose, throat and respiratory tract, while *Hyoscyamus* has a more purely nervous cough with less catarrhal involvement.

Squilla.—Loose, rattling cough with profuse expectoration, associated with sharp, sticking chest pains.

CAPILLARY BRONCHITIS.

Definition.—Capillary bronchitis is an acute catarrhal inflammation of the finer bronchial tubes. It is almost exclusively a disease of infancy, but a few cases are encountered in the aged. It is bilateral and diffuse.

Etiology.—Capillary bronchitis may occur primarily, but is most commonly the result of extension of an acute inflammation of the larger tubes and hence is excited by the same sources of irritation, undue exposure, and predisposition that cause simple acute bronchitis.

3

Pathology.—Capillary bronchitis presents much the same pathological changes as are seen in acute bronchitis of the larger tubes, with this exception that as the capillary bronchioles are so much smaller in calibre and contain no cartilage in their walls the swelling and occlusion when inflamed is much more rapid and complete. The mucous secretion, rich in cellular elements, promptly closes these minute tubes with resulting collapse (atelectasis) or broncho-pneumonia of the air vesicles to which they lead.

Symptoms.—The earlier symptoms are those of a simple acute bronchitis, but with greater intensity, merging into those of respiratory obstruction. There may be a chill or chilliness, followed by fever, restlessness, hacking cough, pain and soreness. As the capillary tubes become obstructed with viscid secretion, the cough grows suffocative, the patient shows marked drowsiness, the dyspnœa is pronounced, the respirations are labored and increased in frequency to forty to eighty per minute. The pulse is weak and rapid, 120 to 150 per minute. Cyanosis develops and is a very prominent symptom, with cool clammy sweat, great restlessness, the respirations grow faint and superficial, the pulse fluttering and uncountable, and the patient sinks into the fatal stupor of deficient blood æration and cardiac failure.

Physical Signs.—Percussion shows an absence of distinct areas of consolidation. Auscultation reveals the subcrepitant rale, which is a fine, moist rale, heard during both inspiration and expiration. Vesicular breathing is diminished or suppressed in localized areas. The earlier rales are sibilant, but they disappear with the formation of secretion and the subcrepitant rales take their place. These are caused by the separation of the agglutinated surfaces of the capillary bronchioles and constitute the diagnostic sign of capillary bronchitis.

Complications.—The most important are atelectasis and broncho-pneumonia.

Diagnosis.—From broncho-pneumonia, with which it is most apt to be confused, the separation is most difficult. Pathologically, the two conditions are distinct, but clinically they are the same. Many recent writers devote only a casual mention to capillary bronchitis from a pathological standpoint, treating it clinically, however, as inseparable from broncho-pneumonia. A broncho-pneumonia must always be associated with a capillary bronchitis, and while it may be possible for a capillary bronchitis to exist very briefly without a broncho-pneumonia, the extension of the inflammation to the air vesicles seems inevitable in so short a time that it is an astute observer who can clearly demonstrate the presence of one without the existence of the other. The strong diagnostic points, as emphasized, of capillary bronchitis as differentiated from broncho-pneumonia are the bilateral distribution of the subcrepitant rales, the absence of distinct areas of consolidation, the patients' age (infancy) and the seeming greater suddenness with which obstruction to respiration, exhaustion, cyanosis and stupor appear and develop. Acute tuberculosis has more sweat, greater variation in temperature, apical involvement, and the presence of the *tubercle bacilli*. Pulmonary œdema is associated with cardiac disease.

Prognosis.—The age of the patient, the extent of respiratory obstruction and the condition of the heart influence the outlook. In general, the prognosis is unfavorable.

Treatment.—The general management of capillary bronchitis and the remedies indicated are the same as in broncho-pneumonia to which the reader is referred.

PLASTIC OR FIBRINOUS BRONCHITIS.

Definition.—May occur as an acute or chronic inflammation of the bronchial tubes and is characterized by the formation of casts of the tubes caused by the unusual fibrinous character of the exudate. These casts are expelled with dyspnœa and cough. This condition should not be confounded with the casts or exudate found in diphtheria, hæmoptysis, phthisis, or the casts of the finer bronchial tubes sometimes met with in pneumonia.

Etiology.—This disease is mostly found in middle life, prior to forty years of age. It is rarely encountered in childhood or infancy and most frequently occurs in males. Its exact etiology is unknown, but it is apparently dependent upon a peculiar constitutional diathesis. Patients affected by plastic bronchitis are usually feeble and anæmic, with latent phthisical tendencies. The spring is the time of the year when it is most prone to occur.

Pathology.—The casts consist mainly of mucin entangling in its meshes various corpuscles, ciliated and cylindrical epithelium, oil globules and granular debris. The casts are usually expelled in a rolled up form, like gelatinous masses, and are generally mixed with free mucus and blood. When carefully unrolled and examined their peculiar formation will appear. In some cases when the larger bronchial tubes are involved the main stem of the cast may be as large as the little finger.

Symptoms.—These are at first those of an acute bronchitis, but as the casts form there will be chilliness or a chill with increased fever and a hard, racking, straining cough. Dyspnœa is present and may be very great if a large tube is the seat of deposit, thus cutting off an extensive tract of lung tissue from respiratory function.

The first expectoration is that of acute bronchitis, but later, after a violent paroxysm, a croupous cast or several of them will be expectorated, relieving the more acute symptoms. The temperature falls and the cough and dyspnœa materially decrease. This may end a simple case, but if a severe one the process may continue and the casts reform in a time, varying from a few hours to several days. The duration of the ordinary acute case is from three or four days to two or three weeks. Diminution in the number and size of the casts with a reduction in the temperature and relief from the dyspnœa and cough marks the progress toward recovery. In the enfeebled if the attack is severe and the area involved extensive, the tendency may be toward a fatal termination. In this event the temperature runs high, the dyspnœa is marked, the pain and cough severe, the respiration rapid, pulse tense, the appearance becomes cyanotic and death takes place from asphyxiation.

The chronic form of plastic bronchitis is secondary to a protracted chronic bronchitis and is associated with symptoms merging with those of the associated pulmonary condition—phthisis or emphysema. The chronic form is marked by remissions for months at a time, during which there will be entire absence of exudation or resulting symptoms.

Physical Signs.—Are those due to obstructed lung tissue. There is an absence of vocal fremitus over the limited area cut off from the respiratory function with diminution in the respiratory sounds. There will be flatness on percussion if this area becomes filled with exudate or collapses, or if it is associated with a phthisical consolidation. After the expulsion of the casts there are moist, whistling rales over the diseased area. Generally speaking, the dry and moist rales of bronchitis attend. Plastic bronchitis often leads to broncho-pneumonia.

Diagnosis.—Is impossible unless the characteristic exudate appears in the sputum. Examine this very thoroughly when the symptoms lead to suspicion of the disease. At first it may appear lumpy, but floated on water it will unfold and reveal its tree-like form. From diphtheria it is differentiated by the fact that in diphtheria the exudate first appears in the pharynx and contains the Klebs-Lœffler bacilli.

General Treatment.—Generally speaking, is the same as in acute or chronic bronchitis. The indication is to remove the bronchial obstruction. Hot steam vapor and inhalations of Menthol, Benzoin, Hypochlorite of Lime, Iodine, or Creosote (one drachm to the pint of boiling water). Emetics are contra-indicated because of the subsequent depression. In chronic cases, a change of climate, going to a warm, equable temperature, or a sea voyage is beneficial. Regulate the general regime and diet.

Remedies.—Of the homœopathic remedies the following are indicated and beneficial:

Kali bichromicum.— Rough, hoarse voice. Hoarse, metallic cough with pain in chest and tightness. Great dyspnœa and oppression, especially at bifurcation of bronchi, as if the mucous membrane were thickened. Expectoration of stringy mucus. Coughs up casts of elastic, fibrinous nature, followed by loud mucous rales and wheezing, rattling cough. Prostration.

Iodine.—Hoarseness, tightness and difficulty of respiration. Wheezing, sawing breathing with dry, barking cough, and finally expectoration of blood-streaked mucus. Emaciation and debility with glandular and catarrhal diathesis.

Bromine.—Scraping and rawness upon respiration with voice hoarse or lost. Croupy cough with sudden paroxysm of suffocation, as if the chest were full of smoke. Weakness and lassitude

Spongia.—Hoarseness with sense of a plug obstructing respiration. Dry, barking, hollow, croupy or asthmatic cough, with wheezing and whistling breathing and great weakness in the chest. Burning, sore pain in chest and bronchi.

Kali iodide.—In saturated solution, three to ten drop doses, administered in water after each meal, is of value in obstinate cases or those where syphilitic taint is known or suspected.

CHRONIC BRONCHITIS.

Definition.—Chronic bronchitis is a chronic catarrhal inflammation of the mucous membrane lining the bronchial tract. It may result as a sequel to repeated attacks of simple acute bronchitis or it may develop as secondary to a variety of morbid conditions.

Etiology.—Climate exerts an important influence. It

is especially prevalent in damp localities and during the winter months. Old people are particularly liable to have it; it is the "winter cough" of old men. The young are less frequently affected, a chronic cough in them usually indicating deeper affections. It develops secondarily in phthisis, emphysema, gout, Bright's disease and various cardiac affections, especially those of the right heart which favor pulmonary stasis.

Morbid Anatomy.—The local changes vary with the duration and extent of the disease and also depend much upon the underlying condition. In the initial stages of an uncomplicated chronic bronchitis the changes are confined to the mucous membrane, but in long lasting cases the submucosa, in fact, the whole tube structure, may become weakened and undergo dilation. At first the mucous membrane becomes thickened, granular, and denuded of epithelium in areas; later these portions undergo atrophy and even ulceration.

Physical Signs.—The chest is distended and its movements limited, this is due to the emphysematous condition. Percussion shows resonance. Auscultation shows a long expiration blended with all kinds of rales, high and sibilant or deep-toned and snoring.

Symptoms.—These vary with the duration and degree of the disease. There is no pain nor soreness. The respiration is wheezy and oppressed. The patient puffs and blows and cough is excited upon exertion, ascending stairs, etc. (due not so much to the bronchitis as the accompanying emphysematous changes). There is no fever except during acute aggravations. The cough varies with the weather and the season. Free and comfortable in the summer, but returns in winter, severe and persistent. In the *dry* form (atrophic stage) the cough is paroxysmal and racking, with scanty expectoration, requiring a great effort to raise it. In the majority of cases there is abundant secretion of muco-purulent type. In the morning hours the cough and expectoration is most troublesome, being the effort to rid the tubes of the night's accumulation. The general health may be fairly good, the only serious tendency being to develop emphysema or bronchiectomy. There are certain cases in which there is an excessive amount of thin, purulent secretion, often greenish, with an offensive odor. This condition is termed *bronchorrhœa* and may last many years without serious effect upon the general health, but is apt to lead to dilatation of the bronchi (bronchiectasis) or to a "*fœtid* bronchitis," with offensive odor and expectoration in thick yellow masses. "Fœtid bronchitis," however, is more apt to be associated with bronchiectasis, abscess, gangrene, or decomposition in phthisical cavities.

Dry bronchitis with atrophy of the tissues is most apt to be found in the aged, especially associated with emphysema. Chronic bronchitis is usually incurable owing to the age and the underlying conditions. It may appear to yield to treatment only to reappear the following winter.

General Treatment.—The general condition, diet, hygiene, etc., are of the utmost importance in treating a case of chronic bronchitis. Such cases, owing to the underlying conditions, present a great variety of symptoms and in prescribing for these cases a careful investigation is necessary to ascertain all associated ailments, and thus in outlining a plan of treatment to cover thoroughly and intelligently the whole morbid situation.

Such cases should seek a warm, equable temperature—
Georgia, South Carolina, Florida, Southern California
and Southern France are particularly desirable. A
change of climate is often very beneficial. The atmosphere should be pure and dry and the altitude moderately
high. Personal hygiene and due regard to nutrition are
highly important. In damp, foggy, changeable weather,
with east winds, the patient should stay indoors. He
should wear woolen underclothing, being careful not to
change to lighter weight too early in the spring and to
resume heavier weight in season in the autumn. Bathing should be frequently and carefully done. Sponging
the face, neck and upper chest, night and morning, with
cold salt and water is particularly advantageous, strength-
ening the locality and inuring the region to exposure.
Digestion should be made good, the diet should be plain
and nutritious. The various malt extracts taken after
eating, and cod liver oil especially, are often very beneficial. If exhaustion is marked or the patient is elderly,
stimulation—whiskey, milk punches or eggnogs, should
be taken. Opiates or sedatives for the cough are rarely
required in chronic bronchitis—expectoration of the accumulated secretion is desirable. having the tendency, as
it does, to decompose and further irritate. But if the
secretion is scanty and the cough incessant, racking and
exhausting, particularly at night, Heroin or Codeiæ, in
tablets, or the formulæ given for acute bronchitis, may
be administered with great relief and advantage. Inhalations of Creosote, Terebene or Eucalyptus are often of
benefit if the secretion is putrid.

Remedies.—In considering these the range is very
extensive, as there are not only the cough and local symp-

toms of the bronchitis per se to relieve, but the associated or underlying condition to consider, and while remedies may at times be necessary exclusively for the bronchitis, better results are often obtained by giving considerable attention to the diseased condition underlying the bronchial lesion.

Ammonium carbonicum.—A tendency to failure of the respiratory and circulatory function. Especially suited to old persons or those much enfeebled, with large accumulation, loud rattling rales and oppression, with little ability or effort to expel secretion. Threatened cardiac and respiratory failure.

Antimonium arsenite.—Chronic cough associated with emphysema and heart affection. Asthmatic breathing, unable to lie down, with profuse expectoration and wheezing or rattling respiration

Antimonium iodatum.—Introduced by Dr. Wm. C. Goodno, and recommended by him as very efficacious in the chronic bronchitis of phthisis or that following influenza. Spasmodic cough, especially morning and evening, free expectoration of muco-purulent matter, loss of strength and flesh with night sweats.

Antimonium tartaricum. --Profuse amount of mucous secretion with inability to expectorate; threatened suffocation with fine mucus rales. Evidence of deficient aeration of the blood, patients lose breath and are cyanotic. Particularly suited to the attacks of old people and infants.

Arsenicum iodatum.—The chronic bronchitis and cough of incipient phthisis. Anæmia and emaciation, anorexia, hyperexia, dyspnœa. Usually a racking, rather dry cough, with purulent expectoration, often blood streaked.

Belladonna.—Dry, paroxysmal cough, nightly aggravation, spasmodic in character and causing flushing of the face and headache, with little or no expectoration. Nervous element.

Carbo vegetabilis.—Bronchitis of old people with little power to expectorate. Exhausted constitutions with torpor of bronchial lining and muscular fibres, profuse mucous expectoration with blue nails and cold extremities.

Drosera.—Severe paroxysmal cough; expectoration of yellow mucus or pus, worse at night; deep hoarse tone to the cough and voice.

Grindelia robusta.—Hard spasmodic cough, fine rales present but scanty mucous expectoration, associated with dyspnœa and emphysema.

Ipecac.—Bronchitis associated with asthma. Spasmodic loose cough, loud mucous rales, free expectoration, with gagging and dyspnœa.

Kali bichromicum.—Torpid and inveterate cases, whistling, wheezing in the chest with burning in the trachea, hoarseness of voice and cough, tough muco-purulent expectoration sometimes fœtid.

Lycopodium.—Valuable remedy for the chronic bronchitis of phthisical subjects, especially associated with the gouty diathesis—flatulence, acid dyspepsia and constipation.

Pulsatilla.—Moist cough with profuse expectoration of yellow or greenish muco-purulent secretion. Especially in anæmic females with uterine irregularities, dyspepsia, bad tasting eructations, erratic pains, chilliness and mental depression.

Phosphorous.—Cough worse night and morning, with huskiness and oppression of chest, small amount of yellow mucous expectoration—thin, feeble subjects.

Rumex crispus.—Dry bronchitis, with hyperæsthesia of larynx and respiratory tract. Cough dry, incessant, hacking, aggravated by pressure, talking, eating, breathing cold air and when lying down.

Spongia.—Cough with tracheal and laryngeal involvement, dry and croupy with rawness in the larynx and hoarseness.

Other remedies to be considered in inveterate cases, are *Sepia*, *Silicia*, the *Calcareas*, *Hepar sulphur*, *Causticum*, *Sanguinaria*, *Sulphur*.

Chininum arsenicosum.—With marked periodicity of the cough when malarial infection is suspected or present.

Kali iodatum.—Obstinate cases showing *Kali* conditions with syphilitic history or taint suspected.

BRONCHIECTASIS.

Definition.—Is a chronic dilatation of the bronchial tubes. It may occur as a congenital anomaly, but this is rare. It most commonly results from any condition in which the muscular walls of the bronchi are weakened or relaxed and not able to withstand strain. Hence it is so often found as a complication of chronic bronchitis where the strain of coughing effort, combined with air pressure and the weight in some cases of the accumulated secretion, cause the walls to give way and dilate; this, occurring time after time in repeated attacks, causes the chronic condition of distention known as bronchiectasis.

Pathology.—The condition may be general or partial and there are two forms, the cylindrical and the sacular. *General* bronchiectasis is always unilateral and usually the result of a chronic interstitial pneumonia. In these cases the bronchial tubes are altered into a series of saculi opening one into another and between which is dense cirrhotic lung tissue. These sacs are lined by smooth membrane and they often lie like large cysts near the lung surface, just beneath the pleura. *Partial* bronchiectasis occurs here and there in one ramification, *i. e.*, one branch or tube of the bronchial tree. Here the dilatation is usually cylindrical, although now and then sacs are found. This condition is most frequently met with in such weakening diseases as phthisis, chronic bronchitis, emphysema, and chronic pleurisy. The retained secretion in all varieties becomes offensive.

Symptoms.—The symptoms are in a great measure those of the underlying conditions, *i. e*—phthisis, chronic bronchitis, emphysema, etc., and hence, in the partial dilatation of these most common causative associate diseases, the diagnosis is exceedingly difficult. Bronchiectasis may be suspected when the patient goes several hours without any cough, and then upon a change of position or any unusual effort suddenly coughs violently and expectorates quite a large amount of secretion, dark in color, purulent in character, acid in reaction and fœtid in odor. Microscopically this accumulated secretion consists of pus cells, mucus and fatty acid crystals.

Physical Signs.—These are not constant nor positive. They vary according to the size and form of the cavities and whether empty or full of accumulation. If the sac cavities are large they may be discovered and often simulate phthisical cavities, except that they are usually found at the base and are unilateral. The diagnosis is not so difficult if the physician has the opportunity to watch the patient over a considerable period of time and sees him frequently. The *character* of the *expectoration* and its expulsion *at such long intervals* is characteristic. There is a similarity between bronchiectasis and phthisis, but in the latter the apices are affected, and both are usually involved; the sputum also contains the tubercle bacilli. Also in phthisis there is a rise of temperature at night, and a sign of most importance is that in phthisis there occurs first dullness *followed* by the cavity while in bronchiectasis we find a cavity followed by the dullness as the latter fills with secretion.

Prognosis.—Victims of bronchiectasis may live a long life, though the bronchiectasis adds to the seriousness of the associated disease. It is, however, a most discouraging condition to treat, as it is chronic of the chronics.

General Treatment.—This should be directed primarily to the initial condition, as it is most foolish to attempt relief of the bronchiectasis per se, without giving attention to its associated disease. As locally antiseptic and healing, the following is excellent: ℞. Guiacol 2 parts, Menthol 10 parts, Ol. Olivii 88 parts. S.—Inject one drachm into the trachea twice daily. Osler highly recommend Creosote inhalations. Stuff the nostrils with cotton and protect the eyes with goggles; put one drachm of Creosote upon water in a saucer and evaporate it over a spirit lamp, inhaling the fumes. Use this for fifteen minutes every other day and increase to using one hour each day. Continue this for three months. Also, Guiacol, Carbolic Acid or Menthol sprays. The general nutrition in these cases is most important and must not be neglected. Cod Liver Oil, Malt Extracts, and stimulation are valuable. Deep breathing; ''coughing down hill,'' *i. e.*, lying on the sofa or bed with the head hanging over the side, lower than the body,—will aid in expelling the accumulated secretion. Bathing the chest with cold salt-water followed by friction, will give tone to the parts. All these points should be attended.

Remedies.—Are mainly those for the underlying condition.

Hepar sulphur.—Strumous diathesis. Glandular and catarrhal tendencies, lack of resistance, sensitive to cold and dampness, cough, hoarseness, large accumulation with tendency to become purulent in character.

Calcarea carbonica.—In giving particular attention to general constitutional condition. Sweats, weakness, glandular enlargements, sensitiveness to climatic changes, chest sensitive and sore. Painless, catarrhal hoarseness with shortness of breath. Cough especially in evening and at night, with profuse expectoration of sweetish mucus.

Sulphur.—General chronicity ; acts so well upon the glandular system and mucous membranes. Hoarseness, weakness, cough with chest pains, emaciated, stooping people, of strumous, psoric type. Valuable as an intercurrent.

Silicia.—Perverted nutrition—scrofulous or rachitic individuals. Chilliness, profuse perspiration, expectoration is thick, yellow, purulent and lumpy.

Stannum iodide.—Is a remedy that most often covers the general totality of this diseased condition. *Iodine* with its peculiar adaptibility to scrofulous people and the aged. Emaciation, exhaustion, chronicity, hepatization of lung tissue with hoarseness, tightness and oppression. Then, *Stannum* with its debilitating sweats and great sense of weakness across the chest, its cough with profuse expectoration of greenish muco-pus of putrid, sweetish and offensive taste. Its nightly aggravation and general phthisical picture. The combination of the two as found in *Stannum iodide* gives a remedy par excellance in bronchiectasis.

Kali bichromicum.—With its offensive, thick, tough expectoration, so difficult to raise, should not be overlooked. Also, the other *Calcareas* (*Iodide* and *Sulphate*) and *Carbo. veg.* are all to be thought of when indicated.

ASTHMA.

Definition.—Asthma is a term often misapplied. It should not be used interchangeably with *dyspnœa* (*i. e.*, renal or cardiac "asthma" is incorrect), but should be applied only to that form of difficult breathing due to spasm of the circular fibres surrounding the bronchial tubes, and to some extent involving the respiratory muscles, and known as bronchial or nervous asthma. Attacks are excited by any local irritation of the bronchial mucous membrane, and in a reflex form, by conditions in other more remote organs.

Etiology.—There are many and various theories as to its causation and all doubtless true, for it is a hydra-headed ailment. It is the consensus of opinion, however, that there is a peculiarly hypersensitive condition of the nervous system, particularly affecting those nerves distributed to the respiratory tract. It is prevalent in certain families; males are more often victims then females. A striking variation of causes induce the paroxysms,

4

change of atmosphere or climate, odors of particular flowers or fruits, emanations from animals, etc., dust, pollen, emotion, uterine or ovarian troubles, abnormal nasal or pharyngeal conditions, certain articles of diet, or indigestion. Chronic cases recur year after year from the least cold or special exciting causes.

Symptoms.—Sometimes there are premonitary signs, as oppression, mental depression, polyuria, chilliness, flatulency, etc. Nocturnal attacks are the most common. The typical attack begins with oppressed and difficult respiration, gradually or rapidly increasing until the accessory muscles of respiration are called into play. Inspiration is short and loud, expiration prolonged and wheezy. The chest becomes distended and barrel-shaped. If the attack is severe, evidence of deficient aeration appear, the face anxious, bedewed with sweat, the pulse grows weak and rapid, hands and feet cold, neck distended and turgescent ; the redness extends to the face which becomes flushed, then blue from cyanosis; the cough is tight, dry and wheezing with scanty tenacious expectoration. Just as appearances begin to look desperate the spasm relaxes (from carbonic acid poisoning), the cough loosens, expectoration becomes freer and the patient sinks back exhausted. The paroxysm may last from a few minutes to several hours. The interval may be from one hour to several weeks.

Physical Signs.—Inspection shows the barrel-shaped chest, the diaphragm is depressed and moves but little. Percussion gives increased resonance due to over-distension. Auscultation reveals all kinds of sibilant and sonorous rales throughout the chest. The sputum consists of small, extra tenacious masses of mucus (called "pearls") floating in thinner mucus. The tenacity is due to super-abundance of mucin. These little pellets if straightened out and examined will be found to be in spiral form. There are many theories as to their formation—but Curschman, who first discovered and described them, considered their shape due to the mucin forming casts of the finer bronchioles which are then expelled by violent coughing and a rotary motion of the ciliated epithelia.

Course.—Severe attacks may repeat at short intervals for several days; in the interval there will be cough and roughened respiration. In the purely nervous type of asthma there may be little cough or other symptoms in the interval. Chronic cases result in chronic bronchitis and emphysema, and these are the lesions left to contend with. Death in a paroyxsm is unknown or at least unrecorded.

General Treatment.—For the immediate relief of a paroxysm use inhalations of chloroform. Sulphate of Morphine, ⅛ to ¼ grain, or Pilocarpine, ⅛ grain, hypodermatically. Nitrite of Amyl., 2–5 drops inhaled from a handkerchief often gives prompt relaxation of the spasm. A cup of strong coffee, a dose of whiskey, the fumes of tobacco, or the application of a mustard plaster, act well in some cases. Inhaling the smoke from burning nitrate of potash with stramonium leaves is an old and efficacious means of relief. Convenient forms of the latter combination in powder, pastiles or cigarettes are to be obtained.

Every case should be carefully examined to ascertain the underlying cause. The influence of climate and occupation ; the personal habits of the patients, especially as to proper rest, sexual excesses or the prejudicial use of alcoholics ; the state of the digestion with special reference to the hepatic and bowel functions or excess of uric acid ; possible nervous influences, notably uterine or ovarian disorders; examine the naso-pharyngeal region for hypertrophied turbinatids or other abnormalities as these are a very frequent causative factor. Cold bathing of the whole body or spinal area is often very beneficial in neurotic cases, also the application of electricity.

Remedies.—Those indicated for the totality of symptoms should be sought. To be especially thought of for the asthma are:

Arsenicum album.—Night attacks of suffocation, cannot lie down, burning chest pains, dry cough, great anxiety, thirst, restlessness, irritability and prostration.

Belladonna.—Nervous excitement, flushed face, throbbing headache, nocturnal aggravation, tight, hard cough, sanguine temperament.

Bryonia.—Hard, dry cough with bronchial soreness and shooting chest pains. Sense of oppression, must sit up to get breath; attack brought on by exposure to wind or from violent exertion.

Cimicifuga racemosa.—Especially helpful in the asthma of rheumatic individuals with muscular aching and nervous irritability. Acts best in mother tincture.

Cuprum arsenite.—Strong evidence of spasmodic character. Violent paroxysm with nausea, vomiting or diarrhœa. Nightly aggravation, great sense of suffocation, patient turns bluish, with thirst, restlessness and cramps in the calves and toes

Grindelia robusta.—Awakes from sleep in attack. Loud wheezing respiration with expectoration of tough mucus, chest filled with coarse rales.

Ipecac.—Asthma with many catarrhal manifestations. Loose, rattling cough, spasmodic in character, with extensive rales throughout the chest. Great difficulty in breathing with sweat, cyanosis, nausea and vomiting; gastric cases with inactive liver and furred tongue.

Kali iodide.—Given empirically in very obstinate cases will very frequently effect a cure where other means have failed. Dose, 5 drops of the saturated solution gradually increased to 20 drops, in water, after each meal.

Lobelia inflata.—Especially suitable to cases of gastric origin. Tight, ringing cough with great dyspnœa. Attack is accompanied by marked sensation of faintness and weakness at the epigastrium with extreme nausea and vomiting.

Nux vomica.—Tearing cough and pharyngeal scraping. Gastric cases or from alcoholic excess. Neurotic, irritable subjects, with distention of the stomach, acidity and constipation.

Quebracho.—Great dyspnœa with cyanosis, compelling the patient to sit up in bed. Acts remarkably in some cases in controlling the paroxysm. Thirty drops of the mother tincture in four ounces of water, teaspoonful doses every fifteen minutes.

Quinine sulphate.—Cases marked by periodicity in malarial regions or suspects.

WHOOPING COUGH.

Definition.—Known also as pertussis and tussis convulsiva. An acute, contagious malady, characterized by a series of convulsive coughs, followed by a long drawn,

spasmodic and audible inspiration. This latter constitutes.
the "whoop" and gives the disease its name.

Etiology.—Whooping cough is contagious and is most
frequently taken by direct contact with one so affected,
but may be contracted from rooms, houses, etc., in which
those suffering from the disease have recently been. It is
most prevalent in the winter and spring months and is
essentially an epidemic disease, though sporadic cases are
occasionally seen.

No age is exempt, though children between two and
ten are by far the most susceptible. In early infancy and
old age it is often a most serious affection. Some persons
seem immune and one attack, as a rule, protects against
another. Epidemics of pertussis frequently follow or
precede epidemics of measles or scarlet fever. Several
investigators have described a bacillus which is invariably
present and is no doubt the specific cause, but is not as
yet fully understood.

Pathology.—Whooping cough has in itself no essential
pathological changes or lesions.

Symptoms.—There is a preliminary or *catarrhal stage*,
lasting from seven to ten days, during which the patient
presents the usual symptoms of an acute cold, slight
fever, lassitude, coryza, injected conjunctiva and bronchial cough. After eight or ten days the catarrhal symptoms improve, but the cough increases in severity and
takes on a paroxysmal character with nightly aggravation. This sequence of symptoms in the presence of epidemic whooping cough makes a tentative diagnosis
possible, though many cases are unsuspected until the
"whoop" establishes the true diagnosis. During the
paroxysmal stage the symptoms are characteristic. The

child seems to have a warning sensation of fear or dread, with some oppression or dyspnœa, and runs at once to the parent or nurse for aid and support. The paroxym consists of a series of rapid expiratory coughs, increasing in intensity and terminating with a long drawn, crowing inspiration, which constitutes the "whoop." The paroxysm results in the expectoration of a variable quantity of tenacious, glairy mucus, which is expelled by a combined gagging and coughing effort. If the paroxyms are severe and frequent vomiting is quite usual. During the attack, which lasts from one-half to five minutes, very little air enters the lungs with resulting appearances of deficient aeration. The face becomes swollen and turgescent, the veins are distended, the eyeballs red and protruded. Suffocation seems imminent when the crowing inspiration relieves the situation. In mild cases there may be only three or four paroxysms daily, while in severe cases they may occur every half hour. The attacks are excited by crying, eating, laughing or exertion. The acute spasmodic stage lasts from two to four weeks and then very gradually subsides by diminution in severity and frequency of the paroxysms. The recovery, however, is protracted.

Complications.—The violence of the paroxyms of cough frequently induces epistaxis or conjunctional hæmorrhage and occasionally hæmoptysis. A small superficial ulcer will be found under the tongue in about one-third of the cases. It is due to friction of the frænum against the teeth during coughing. If the attack is severe the frequent vomiting becomes a serious factor in inducing anæmia and exhaustion. Bronchitis is usually present. The most frequent and serious complication is broncho-pneumonia with atelectasis.

Among the less frequent complications are pleurisy, pneumo-thorax, heart strain, and convulsions from cerebral engorgement.

Diagnosis.—During the catarrhal stage the diagnosis is important but difficult. A series of rapid convulsive coughs with tendency to gagging, the age of the child and a nightly aggravation are suggestive. In the paroxysmal stage the "whoop" and other evidences make the diagnosis an easy matter.

Prognosis.—In uncomplicated cases the prognosis is good, but an associated broncho-pneumonia makes the outlook very grave. The prognosis is influenced by the strength of the patient and the violence of the disease. In England whooping cough ranks third in diseases as a cause of fatality among children.

General Treatment.—A child with pertussis should not be permitted to associate with any but the immune, and delicate children should, if possible, be removed from a school or neighborhood when the disease is prevalent. The idea so often advanced by ignorant parents that it is best to expose a child at once to all those infectious diseases, as "it must have them sooner or later any way," is most pernicious and must be combatted. Whooping cough must be regarded as contagious so long as the "whoop" is present and the cough is paroxysmal. Parents should be warned of the serious nature of the disease. The patient should wear suitable underclothing and avoid undue exposure. Fresh air and a good nutritious diet are important. Moderate outdoor exercise may be enjoyed; avoiding violent exertion. Rectal enemata of nourishment and rest in bed may be necessary if the attack is severe and vomiting is frequent. Change of climate is beneficial in severe and protracted cases. The patient should be carefully watched during convalescence for complications. So many palliatives are recommended that it is doubtful if one possesses virtue over another. In cases of moderate intensity they are not necessary. In severe cases the inhalation for ten minutes several times daily of the steam from a one per cent. solution of Carbolic acid, Terebene, Creosote, Guaiacol or Eucalyptol, in a suitable atomizer or open dish, may modify the paroxysms. The dry vapor of either of the four last of these diluted one-half with alcohol may be used carefully from an inhaler or handkerchief with benefit. The author has found inhalations of the steam arising from a small teaspoonful of Hypochlorite of Lime (common bleaching powder) in a pint of hot water or the following, R. Tr. Benzoin ʒi, Menthol grs. x, boiling water ʒxvi, soothing and beneficial. One of the most efficacious means of modifying and shortening the disease is to dress the patient each morning in fumigated clothing, and after removal thoroughly fumigate the sleeping room for five or six hours daily with sulphur fumes, the patient returning each night to sleep in the room after it has been well aired. Excellent results have been obtained from this method.

Remedies.—*Belladonna.*—In the beginning or in severe attacks, frequent violent paroxysms of hard dry cough, worse at night, with flushed face, eyes swollen and conjunctiva injected. Child cries after cough which induces headache, involuntary micturition, or even nose bleed. Nervous twitching or convulsion.

Castanea vesca.—A dry, ringing, violent, convulsive cough, especially if associated with intestinal catarrh and a longing for warm drinks.

Corallium rubrum.—Spasms of dry, suffocative cough, so rapid and violent that the child loses its breath and turns blue in the face, followed by great exhaustion and hawking of mucus or even blood.

Cuprum metallicum.—Violent and long-continued paroxysms of cough, completely exhausting the patient. Child becomes rigid and the face turns purple. Paroxysm is followed by vomiting and is relieved by a swallow of water.

Drosera.—A favorite remedy because so often indicated. Paroxysms of spasmodic, dry cough, following each other in rapid succession, threatening suffocation and resulting in retching or vomiting, with mucus expectoration or bleeding from the nose and mouth. Deep, hoarse voice and hoarseness worse at night. Harrowing, titillating cough.

Ipecac.—Suffocative, incessant and violent cough, the child becoming stiff and blue in the face. There is constriction of the chest and much rattling of mucus. The cough causes nausea and vomiting, with epistaxis or hæmoptysis. An excellent remedy, especially with much bronchial secretion, nausea and gagging

Magnesia phosphorica.—Asthmatic oppression. Dry, tickling, spasmodic cough, with chilliness, flatulent colic and bloated abdomen. Symptoms relieved by warmth. Especially suited to weak, exhausted subjects.

Mephitis.—Suffocative feeling, spasmodic cough, so violent patient must be raised up, cannot exhale, gets blue in the face. Attacks especially at night; mucus rales in the chest. Acts best in 1x to 3x.

Naphthalin.—Long-continued paroxysms of convulsive cough, cannot get breath; with bladder irritation. Has been much used in this affliction with good results, in lower potencies.

III.

Diseases of the Lungs.

NOTE.—Pneumonic Fever and Tuberculosis are properly classified as general infectious diseases, but are here given because their most usual and serious manifestations occur in the lungs. The chapter on Tuberculosis in general is introduced to cover the subject more comprehensively before describing its pulmonary lesions.

III.

DISEASES OF THE LUNGS.

LOBAR PNEUMONIA.

Known also as croupous or fibrinous pneumonia; Pneumonitis; Pneumonic Fever; the "lung fever" of our forefathers.

Definition.—An acute infectious disease characterized by an inflammation of the lungs, the development of a specific organism—the diplococcus pneumoniæ (or micrococcus lanceolatus), the filling of the alveoli with a dense fibrinous exudate; a general systemic toxæmia of varying intensity, and a fever which terminates abruptly by crisis.

Secondary infective processes may involve the pericardium, the endocardium, the pleura, or the cerebrospinal meninges.

Occurrence.—Pneumonia is the most widespread and fatal of all acute diseases. In the United States during 1890, the last census year, there died of it 76,496, a death rate of 186.94 to every 100,000 population. In Chicago it has replaced consumption as the chief cause of mortality and this seems to be the general tendency in other localities. The predisposing influence of influenza doubtless has much to do with this increase. In the last ten years the death rate was 18.03 to 10,000 population, against

12.36 in the preceding ten years. The admission of pneumonia cases to hospitals has doubled in the last few years.

Etiology.—Cold and exposure have always been regarded as important factors in the causation of pneumonia, and there is no doubt that the disease attacks its victims in a vast majority of cases after undue exposure, a chilling, damp feet, or follows a few days of simple coryza. In the light of present knowledge we understand, however, that exposure is only an exciting or predisposing cause in pneumonia by lowering the bronchial and pulmonary resistance.

Climate.—Is not an important factor, as the disease is found in hot and cold countries about alike.

Season—Exerts a great influence, by far the greater number of cases occurring in the winter and spring months, especially in February and March, due doubtless to the changeableness and rawness of the prevailing winds.

Age.—From the first to the sixth year the tendency is marked, then diminishes to the fifteenth, but subsequently increases rapidly with age.

Sex.—Males suffer more frequently than females; this may be due to their being more often subject to severe exposure. Census of 1890 shows 42,739 males, 33,757 females.

Race.—Pneumonia is more fatal in the colored than in the white races.

Social Condition.—It is more prevalent in cities than in the rural districts. New comers and immigrants are less frequently attacked than natives.

Personal Condition.—Any mode or habit of life that tends to debilitate or reduce the general tone predisposes; the most potent source of fatality is alcoholism. Strong healthy people are, however, not exempt.

Recurrence.—One attack strongly predisposes to another, and some persons pass through several attacks. One man, Benj. Rush by name, had it 28 times, and so far is the proud bearer of the record.

Trauma.—Bruises and other injuries to the chest occasionally cause pneumonia, probably acting as the exciting cause. Those who work in factories filled with dust, also are prone to the disease.

Bacteriology.—The fact that pneumonia was an infectious disease was recognized long before its bacteriology was understood. Its mode of outbreak is like that of other infectious diseases; it frequently occurs in endemic form, attacking one person after another in crowded houses, schools, prisons, barracks, etc. Its clinical course is that of all acute infectious diseases, self-limited and running a regular course with crisis, as in the other infectious diseases. As in these the constitutional disturbance is many times out of all proportion to the local lesion, a slight pneumonia of the apex often showing profound general toxæmia and *vice versa* (as also in diphtheria, scarlatina, typhoid, etc.). The essential bacteria of lobar pneumonia is the " *diplococcus pneumoniæ*," which is found very plentifully in the sputum, and has also been repeatedly demonstrated present in large numbers in the fluid drawn from the hepatized lobe with an aspirating syringe. As its name indicates, the pneumococcus is found in pairs; it is elliptical in form and encapsulated. Its usual point of attack is the lungs, but it is often widely distributed, being found in the pleura, endo- and pericardium, cerebro-spinal meninges, nose and accessory cavities as well as in the breast milk in nursing women suffering with pneumonia. These germs leave the body chiefly by way of the sputum and retain their vitality a long time. In view of the bacteriology, all other causes of pneumonia are merely the exciting ones.

Pathology and Morbid Anatomy.—The course of pneumonia may be divided into three stages:

The Stage of Engorgement or Congestion.—In this the affected lobe becomes engorged with blood, the epithelium lining the alveoli becomes red, turgescent, the interlobular and subpleural connective tissue is swollen and the capilliaries tortuous and surcharged with blood. Air still enters the inflamed area, but the tissue becomes heavier, darker red in color, even purple; it pits and crepitates upon pressure, but a portion of it thrown in water will still float. The alveoli begin to fill with a thin serum, reddish and stained from the presence of exfoliated epithelium and exuded red blood corpuscles.

The Stage of Consolidation or Red Hepatization.—In this stage the air cells become stopped with a tough fibrinous exudate consisting of fibrin, red and white blood corpuscles and desquamated epithelium. No air now enters the alveoli, the lung is dark red, like liver in appearance, does not crepitate on pressure and sinks when thrown into water. The dark red color is due to the engorged capillaries and to the exuded red blood corpuscles; the alveoli filled with these give to the lung a granular appearance when a section is made. This is known also as the stage of "red hepatization."

The Stage of Resolution or Grey Hepatization.—In this stage the lung presents much the same characteristics as the second stage, *i. e.*, heaviness and solidity, lack of crepitation and liver-like consistence, the tissue, however, begins to take on a lighter color. This is due to the presence of the firm exudate pressing the contents from the capillaries, the pouring out of leucocytes into the exudate and their destruction of the red blood cells. As this stage progresses the lung grows softer because of the disappearance of the red blood corpuscles and the gradual liquification of the fibrin. A more advanced stage of the grey hepatization is a condition of diffuse purulent infiltration in which the softened exudate becomes rich in pus cells. Having undergone these various changes the aveolar contents, in favorable cases, gradually disappear by expectoration and absorption. In some cases, in which one lobe after another is attacked, the various stages may be seen coincident in the same lung. In cases not leading to prompt resolution the amount of fibrin in the exudate increases, the various cells disappear, new connective tissue is formed, the diseased portion of the lung contracts and a condition of chronic interstitial pneumonia results. Cases of apparently acute pneumonia going into a rapid tubercular degeneration were probably tubercular from the start.

Other Organs.—Aside from the pathological changes in the lung during the course of lobar pneumonia other organs suffer inflammatory changes. The most frequent is *pleurisy;* this is an almost constant accompaniment to pneumonia, hence the popularity of the designation "pleuropneumonia." The association of the pleuritis depends upon the location of the pneumonic inflammation. If it is central pleurisy is infrequent, but if extending to the surface, which it usually does, pleurisy occurs because of contiguity of the serous membranes and simple extension of the inflammatory process. The *blood* shows but littie change, except for the increase of fibrin. Anæmia is

5

not common, as the duration of the disease is too brief. *Endocarditis* and less frequently *pericarditis* occur more often than is generally supposed. Endocarditis occured in 16 out of 100 cases examined post-mortem. *Meningitis* occasionally is a complication. It is especially apt to be present when there is an ulcerative endocarditis. Less common are changes in the liver, spleen and gastro-intestinal tract. Abscess or gangrene occurs as a rarity in the lung in case of imperfect resolution.

Symptoms.—There is, as a rule, no pronounced period of invasion or prodromic symptoms. The patient may have experienced slight feeling of malaise and depression with some mild symptoms of a catarrhal nature. But in lobar pneumonia, more marked than in any other disease, the

Invasion is sharp, decided and severe. The patient is seized without warning while at work, during sleep or other unexpected time, with a pronounced and severe chill. Even during the chill the thermometer shows the fever is rising. Shortly after the onset the patient shows flushed features, headache, and general pains. Within a few hours a sharp chest pain develops of an agonizing character due to the associated pleurisy. A short, dry, painful, hacking cough begins with scanty *rust colored* expectoration. The temperature rises to 104°–105°, and by the second or third day the patient presents a very characteristic appearance. He lies flat in bed, usually on the affected side, as the pressure eases the pain and gives the well side more play in respiration. The breathing is hurried and labored, the alæ nasi distended with each inspiration and a short expiratory grunt accompanies each expiration. The cough is frequent, dry, racking and causing sharp pain, so that he winces and holds his side, with the characteristic *rusty* and *very tenacious* expectoration. The face is deeply flushed, especially upon the cheeks, with herpes about the lips. The skin is hot and dry, the eyes bright and shining, and the expression very anxious. The temperature is usually 104° to 106°, the pulse full and bounding, and its ratio out of proportion to the rapid respiration. There are all the. signs of consolidation in the lungs, bronchial breathing and crepitant rales. In from seven to ten days the temperature falls with a rapid return to a sense of comfort. This is a description of a typical case. Now to consider the symptoms in detail:

The Fever.—Rises rapidly after the chill and may reach its acme in twelve hours, but is usually at its height by the second day. Having reached 104° to 105° it remains very constant with morning remissions of from 1 to 2 degrees. In the aged and inebriates the temperature runs lower than in children or the robust. There are rare cases with a very low degree of fever. During the chill, especially in old people, the shock may be so severe that unconsciousness or collapse symptoms may appear. The day of the crisis is variable. In some cases it may occur as early as the third day, while in others it may be delayed until the twenty-first day. These tedious cases, however, are usually caused by an extension of the inflammation to new areas or complications in other organs. The usual time for the crisis is the seventh or eighth day and it should be expected at that time. The very rapid fall of temperature in pneumonia is striking. In most cases it only takes about twelve hours. The fever will fall from 104° or 105° to normal or below, accompanied by a profuse perspiration; the pain, cough, respiratory distress all disappear promptly and the patient falls into a quiet, natural sleep. The peculiarity of it is that all this occurs without any perceptible change in the condition in the lung itself. In some instances the temperature falls so rapidly, occupying only five or six hours, to normal or even lower (to 96° or 95°), accompanied by vomiting, diarrhœa, profuse cold sweat, that a condition of collapse maintains. In other cases two or three days are required for the return to normal, this is particularly true since influenza made its appearance. There may be a slight rise for two or three hours before the crisis, and again after the crisis there may be a slight rise to 101° or 102°. This is doubtless due to contamination of the blood by the absorption of the exudation. A pronounced rise of temperature to 102° or 104° after defervescence indicates that the disease has invaded a new lobe, or the occurrence of pleurisy, empyema, gangrene or abscess. If the fever lasts until the twelfth day, the decline is by lysis; this is especially apt to occur in the case of children. If resolution is protracted the temperature may maintain over a period of several weeks. In debilitated persons a rapid fall sometimes precedes death and should not be mistaken for the crisis. Usually, however, a rapid rise precedes dissolution.

Pain.—Is due to the attending pleuritis. Absent in central pneumonia, but marked in inflammations near the surface. Very sharp and distressing usually just below nipple of affected side—also found in axilla and posteriorly under the scapula.

Respiration.—Difficult and rapid, out of ratio to the pulse, usually runs from 30 to 40, while the pulse may be only 100 to 120. May be as high 60 or 80. Inspiration is short and expiration accompanied by a grunt, while the chest movements on affected side are limited voluntarily to avoid pain.

Pulse.—Heart failure is a marked tendency in pneumonia. It may develop rapidly or slowly, and appear as early as the third day or during the crisis or thereafter. Due to the effort of the heart to supply the system with oxygen, impeded by the occluded lung, high fever, and also to specific poisoning of the cardiac muscle by the bacteria. In most favorable cases the pulse is 100 to 110. Rate of 120 to 130 is a cause for apprehension.

Cough.—Is hard, frequent and restrained, accompanied by great pain and after first few hours with a characteristic viscid, blood tinged and very tenacious expectoration. In low types of the disease the expectoration may be dark fluid, resembling prune juice. In some forms, especially in drunkards or the aged, the cough and expectoration may be absent.

Gastro-intestinal Symptoms.—Vomiting is quite common early in the disease, especially in children. Tongue is usually white and furred, but in some cases or late in the disease may be dry and brown. Constipation is the rule with anorexia. The spleen and liver may be enlarged, the latter, from the engorged right heart.

Urine.—Presents early the usual fibrile symptoms of high color, increased specific gravity and acidity, with traces of albumin. The characteristic and important diagnostic sign of pneumonia (unlike pleurisy with effusion or empyema) is the diminution or absence of chlorides in the urine.

Skin.—Herpetic eruption is very usual, especially about the lips. Profuse sweating at and immediately following the crisis is the rule. The cheeks, particularly during the height of the disease, are markedly flushed, especially the cheek on the affected side.

Cerebral Symptoms.—Convulsions frequently usher in the disease in children. Headache is very common. As a rule delirium is not usual in pneumonia, but may develop in a low or severe type of the disease, especially in those with unsound kidneys and drunkards. In some cases it becomes maniacal and in others, particularly in children, so resembles the symptoms of meningitis that the latter is diagnosed and the pneumonia overlooked. Mental aberration may continue into and after convalescence.

Physical Signs. — *First Stage.*—Respiratory movements over the affected side are limited according to the degree of pain. Slight percussion, dulness gradually increasing, with diminished respiratory sound (due to voluntary restraint) and broncho-vesicular breathing and some sub-crepitant rales. The crepitant rale is the most important diagnostic sign in pneumonia and is due to the separation by the ingress of air of the walls of the aveoli, which are adhered together by the viscid secretion. It is heard at the close of the inspiratory act and is more pronounced after coughing or after deep inspiration. This rale disappears as the cells fill with exudate and reappears as air again enters the lung with progressing resolution. The vocal and other signs of consolidation appear and increase toward the close of this stage.

Second Stage.—In this stage the air cells become filled with firm, tenacious exudate. Respiratory movement is much more limited than during first stage, then it was due to pain and was voluntary, now it is due to the fact that no air enters the consolidated lobe. As a natural result movement of the well side is much increased. Percussion shows dulness, increasing to flatness over diseased area. Palpation gives increased vocal fremitus. In no disease is bronchial breathing so marked with both inspiration and expiration. Bronchophony is also present. It must be remembered that pleural effusion reaching a line above the pneumonic lobe will alter the physical signs, all becoming less distinct.

Third Stage.—The physical signs recede in reverse order. Bronchophony gives way to vocal resonance. Bronchial breathing to that of vesicular character, the crepitant rale reappears mixed with the coarser rales of exudate in the smaller tubes (the "Rale Redux"). Dulness gradually shades into resonance, expansion of the lung takes place and respiratory movement returns. Resolution may take place slowly and so the physical signs of consolidation prolong for some weeks.

In Children.—Pneumonia in childhood is accompanied by more symptoms of the nervous system. Headache, delirium, or stupor are more often present. Convulsions often occur, especially at the onset of the disease, but may appear later during its course, followed by delirium or semi-consciousness, with voluntary urination and defæcation. This may lead to error in the diagnosis. The presence of cough with short, labored, grunting respiration, which is very rapid (50 to 80 per minute), should lead to a careful examination of the chest, lest a pneumonia be mistaken for one of the various forms of meningitis.

Varieties.—*Epidemic* pneumonia often shows peculiarities. In one epidemic typhoid symptoms may be prominent, in another heart complications, in another cerebral, another gastro-intestinal features, etc. In the pneumonias consequent upon the influenza of recent years, the onset is more insidious and the mortality high in those past middle life. Cases secondary to existing cardiac or renal disease are usually rapid and severe, with tendency to pulmonary œdema, abscess or gangrene. In inebriates the symptoms are often masked by the cerebral manifestations; these cases usually have a low range of temperature and the prognosis is unfavorable. In the aged pneumonia is adynamic, with low temperature; pain, cough and expectoration moderate, *i. e.*, the general symptoms do not keep pace with what we would expect from the lesion. Double pneumonia is rare and differs from the unilateral only in seriousness. Central pneumonia does not present physical signs as clearly as one extending to the periphery. Epidemic pneumonia often is peculiar in attacking many persons under one roof, as in one house, prison, school, or barracks, a clear indication of its infective nature.

Complications.— *Pleuritis* is present in a large majority of cases and is inevitable when the pneumonic inflammation involves the lung surface. It usually appears early in the disease with quite copious exudation, peculiarly rich in fibrin. Other cases appear later during the course of the disease by extension of inflammation; these show less exudation. In all cases the pneumococcus is present in the pleuritic fluid.

In pneumonia frequently a pleurisy will develop on the side opposite than that affected by the pneumonia. In such a case with effusion care should be taken not to mistake it for a double pneumonia.

Empyema has been quite frequently seen, especially since the prevalence of influenza. A hacking cough, short, labored breathing, restricted chest-motion, hectic fever and prostration, *after* defervesence has taken place and the patient *should* be recovering, should lead to a careful physical examination. The exploring needle may be needed to decide the question.

Endocarditis is a frequent complication, especially if there were previously existing valvular disease. It is of malignant type due to the infection of the pneumococcus and usually occurs in the left heart. Its discovery is difficult, as the physical signs are usually negative. It may be suspected with more or less certainty if embolism occurs, if sepsis appears, or meningitis is present.

Pericarditis of an acute type is of frequent occurrence and makes a serious complication. It is especially found in the young. The exudation is mostly fibrinous. There may be no local symptoms, owing to the preponderance of the pneumonia, but pain, rapid respiration and a feeble, accelerated pulse, should lead to a careful investigation of the precordial region.

Meningitis is found in 8 per cent. of fatal cases. It usually appears during the height of the pneumonia, but may develop earlier or later. Its diagnosis during life is difficult, owing to the fact that in such cases it usually affects the convexity of the brain. It may be suspected in profound types of pneumonia, with delirium or coma and eye symptoms, paralysis, and bladder and bowel incontinence.

Bronchitis.—A general bronchitis may be present. Evidenced by the character of the cough, breathing and rales, which are bilateral. Especially in the pneumonias following influenza.

Pulmonary œdema may develop in feeble individuals or those with diabetes, chronic nephritis, etc. Recognized by bubbling rales, frothy watery expectoration, cyanosis, oppressed breathing, anxiety and coma. Bilateral.

Paralysis — paraplegic or hemplegic—may occur, especially in low types of the disease with brain symptoms predominating. May develop early or late in the disease.

Jaundice may set in at any time, particularly in certain epidemics, probably due to an infective catarrhal process in liver.

Diagnosis.—In the majority of cases diagnosis of lobar pneumonia is not difficult—the severe chill, the external appearance, the sputa, the physical signs, the onset—all are characteristic in the average case. In *children* the symptoms frequently resemble those of meningitis, and again pneumonia may be present without cerebral symptoms or even others which would indicate the trouble to be in the lungs, emphasizing the importance of a careful physical examination if the symptoms make it possible that pneumonia exists. Pleurisy with effusion in children sometimes so resembles the pneumonic fever that the exploring needle may have to be resorted to to make a diagnosis.

Broncho-pneumonia is bilateral, and owing to the bronchial tubes being occluded, the respiration is more labored, the tendency to cyanosis greater, there is more cough and expectoration, which is not rusty, with bronchial rales, the onset is more gradual and generally follows a previous bronchitis, whooping cough, or measles. Pneumonia occurring in the aged, in drunkards, during the course of Bright's disease, diabetes, chronic heart disease, etc., without marked chest or other characteristic symptoms may often be undetected. The character of the respiration and the temperature are the best indications, and in all such cases any new symptoms should excite suspicion and call for thorough and frequent examinations of the chest.

Prognosis.—In healthy individuals, not in the extremes of life, with good care and treatment the prognosis is favorable and they usually recover fully. In the aged, the debauched, and in victims of various chronic maladies, especially those of the heart and kidneys, the mortality is disastrous. The mortality in those over sixty is over 50 per cent. The general average mortality is from 12 per cent. to 40 per cent., varying with epidemics and locality, being higher in the Southern States. Complications exert a grave influence, especially meningitis and endocarditis. Death is due to cardiac failure or the general toxæmia, not to asphyxia. The temperature is a significant omen. A temperature of 104° is favorable, but if it continues to rise after the fourth day it is unfavorable. A low temperature range, if the pulse and respiration correspond, is favorable. A pulse of 120 or over, especially if it is thready, compressible or intermittent is of grave account. Offensive expectoration, or if "prune juice" in character, shows deterioration of blood and tissues, or possibly gangrene. Tracheal rales, especially with inability to expectorate, usually portend death and indicate pulmonary œdema. Cases beginning with severe gastro-intestinal symptoms show double the mortality of those beginning with chill. Rapid development of consolidation, a large amount of frothy expectoration, respiration rate over fifty, increased rapidity of pulse and rise of temperature after the seventh day, delirium throughout the twenty-four hours, are each and all unfavorable signs.

General Treatment.—The room should be large and kept well ventilated and at a temperature of 68° to 70°. If the cough is dry, hacking, or harsh, the atmosphere may be made humid by steam from a pan of water on the stove. The patient should be kept at perfect rest on a firm mattress and not permitted to rise to the sitting position for any purpose whatever. No company or other excitement should be permitted. Carefully conducted sponge bathing with warm soap and water or alcohol and water is necessary and beneficial. An abundance of pure water should be administered. This is very important. It may be flavored with lemon, orange, tamarinds, or grape juice. The diet should be generally liquid, light, easily digestible and nutritious, and given at regular intervals and in stated quantities. It may consist of milk, peptonized or with lime water, junket, animal broths, cereal gruels, very soft or *raw* eggs, gelatin, café-au-lait, boiled or baked custards, etc.

The bowels should be kept regular by enemas, if necessary, and at the outset if there is a history or evidence of torpidity, a mild laxative should be used—a Seidlitz powder, a glass of effervescent Citrate of Magnesia, or Cascara sagrada. The bladder should be watched lest in low conditions retention of urine be over looked and do injury.

Local Applications.—In simple cases without severe pain the pneumonia jacket is an excellent measure for protection. If the pleuritic pain is severe, hot flaxseed poultices or hot fomentations give comfort and are of benefit. Ice bags are used by some, especially in Germany, for the same purpose. The hot water bag may be sufficient. It is doubtful if these local measures have any direct beneficial effect on the disease itself as each has its devotees and all claim good results—so let experience and common sense decide which should be used.

Stimulation.—If the pulse remains good, prostration is not marked and the digestive power is not impaired, no alcoholic stimulant may be needed throughout the course of the disease, and as a general proposition it is best to do without it if not indicated.

Feeble digestion will improve under small quantities given with the food (ʒi to iv in milk). Alcohol in these cases has no effect upon the temperature. In fact, large quantities of stimulant are often required in pneumonia, and, if so, are well tolerated, producing no symptoms of alcoholism. In threatened heart failure alcohol is invaluable, or if the general prostration is marked it should be given. Whiskey or brandy are the most suitable and may be given in doses varying from two to eight drachms every two to four hours. One drachm every hour acts well in some cases. In seriously threatened cardiac or general collapse champagne given freely is of great value and well tolerated.

Heart failure.—Must be promptly combatted if it threatens during the course of pneumonia. It is indicated by apathy, cold extremities, clammy sweat, feeble, thready pulse, cyanosis, and quick gasping respiration. Whiskey or brandy, as already mentioned, in doses of two to eight drachms every one to three hours. Oxygen as a cardiac and pulmonary restorative may be administered at intervals for several days to tide over the critical period. Give for from five to fifteen minutes at the beginning of each hour, or continuously for several hours if the patient's condition is imminently dangerous. Strychnine, Nitrate or Sulphate is the most reliable tonic stimulant to the cardiac muscle and should be given in doses of from $\frac{1}{100}$ to $\frac{1}{50}$ of a grain, by mouth or hypodematically, every three to four hours, in cardiac **exhaustion** or threatening failure. Nitro-Glycerine, $\frac{1}{100}$ to $\frac{1}{200}$ of a grain, every three to six hours, more a stimulant, transitory in action, valuable in a crisis because of its promptness, but Strychnine is more to be depended upon for regular and continued use. Digitalis, the tincture, in five to ten drop doses every one to four hours in those cases with feeble intermittant pulse and threatening pulmonary œdema.

Remedies.—*Aconite.*—Called for at the onset and during the first stage. Chill, followed by high fever, flushed face, thirst, restlessness, anxiety, general pains, hacking cough, with rusty expectoration.

Antimonium tartaricum.—During resolution, fine crepitant and subcrepitant rales throughout the formerly consolidated area, with loose cough and difficult expectoration of muco-purulent type. The patient is weak, with cool, clammy skin, perspiration, quick, feeble pulse. Of great value in old people or infants when resolution threatens suffocation with exhaustion, inability to expectorate, cyanosis, threatened pulmonary paralysis or œdema.

Bryonia alba.—Second stage of the disease when pleurisy is well marked. Fever, frontal headache, thirst, hectic flush. Breathing is oppressed, short and panting, because of intense pleural pain. Cough short and suppressed, with scanty rusty expectoration.

Ferrum phosphoricum.—The attack is not so sharp, chill not so severe, fever not so high, less restlessness and thirst, tendency to apathy, more bronchitis. Sputum more rusty, or even bloody. Not of value if pluritis is a marked feature. Especially valuable in weak, anæmic persons, those debilitated by previous chronic disease, secondary pneumonia, or when reaction is poor.

Hepar sulphur.—Stage of resolution; husky, weak voice and hoarse, loose cough; rattling rales; cool, moist skin, sensitive to the least exposure. Patients of weak, strumous type.

Iodine.—Very efficacious in condition of complete hepatization, particularly if on the left side. Cough dry and hard with sense of constriction, high fever with great oppression and rapid respiration. Especially in scrofulous subjects.

Kali bichromicum. — During resolution with tough, tenacious expectoration, difficult to raise, loud, coarse rales, prostration, sweat, furred tongue, sluggish people.

Phosphorus.—Enjoys greater repute than any other remedy in the stage of hepatization. Weight and oppression of the chest, embarrassment of respiration which is short and panting. Cough causing pain in the chest, worse evening and at night, with difficult, scanty expectoration of tenacious rust-colored mucus. General hectic appearance, fever and prostration. Severe cases, "typhoid" pneumonia.

Sulphur.—Where resolution is delayed or incomplete, as an intercurrent and to aid in making a good and complete recovery.

Veratrum viride.—For very intense cases setting in with violent chill, very active congestion and delirium, followed by high fever, with full, hard bounding pulse. May be given in one or two drop doses every half to one hour until arterial excitement subsides.

In addition to the classical remedies mentioned consider also the following: In the pneumonia of old people *Ammon. carb.*, *Antim. ars.*, *Carbo veg.* In low types of the disease with typhoid appearances, "prune juice," expectoration, etc., *Bapt.*, *Lach.*, *Rhus tox.* For nervous symptoms, *Bell.*, *Hyos.*, *Stram.*

In neglected or unresolved cases, *Hepar sulph.*, *Lycop.*, *Silicia*, *Sulphur.* To aid in convalescenc, *China*, *Chin. arsen.*, *Ferr. Arsen.*

TUBERCULOSIS.

General Consideration.

Definition.—An infectious disease due to the presence of the bacillus tuberculosis and characterized by the formation of nodular lesions or diffuse areas of tuberculous infiltration which undergo caseation or sclerosis and later may ulcerate or in some cases calcify.

History.—The word "tubercle" had long been used to indicate nodular growths, but it was not until the early part of the 19th Century that Bayle and Lænnec employed the term specifically to describe the lesions of tuberculosis. In 1839 Schönlein first applied the term "tuberculosis" to indicate a definite disease. In 1865 Villemin demonstrated that tuberculosis could be communicated to animals by inoculation. While tuberculosis had been generally regarded as contagious and heredi-

tary from the earliest times, without knowledge of its
cause, it remained for Koch, after a series of brilliant
and scientific experimentation to isolate and demonstrate
in 1882 the bacillus as its definite cause.

Etiology.—*Zoölogy.*—Tuberculosis is rarely found in
animals living in a natural state. Cold blooded animals
are practically exempt. Among domestic animals it is
common, especially in bovines. This fact is important
as beef and milk form so important articles of food.
Horses and sheep are very rarely attacked. It is common in pigs, but less so in this country than abroad.
Dogs, cats, rabbits and guinea pigs are not prone to the
disease in a natural state and when attacked usually get it
from a diseased master and are very susceptible to inoculation.

Man. Tuberculosis is the most universal and fatal
scourge of the human race. One-seventh of all deaths
are due to it. It is more prevalent in large cities or
where the population is massed together. In the United
States 150,000 die annually of it and 1,050,000 (or 1 in
60) are infected with it.

Geographical position exerts less importance than altitude. More prevalent in the temperate zone, but is found
in all. In high altitudes the death rate from tuberculosis
is low.

Race is of less importance than the conditions under
which the various peoples live, as to exposure and sanitation. In our own country the Irish and Negro are
very prone to the disease, while Hebrews are relatively
immune. Dr. Frank Kraft claims that bald-headed men
are well-nigh exempt.

Decrease.—During the past twenty years there has

been a decided decrease in the prevalence of the disease, owing to its infective nature being better understood with consequent improved sanitation and hygiene.

The Bacillus.—This appears as a short fine rod, often slightly curved, with the length of one-half the diameter of a red blood corpuscle. Sometimes shows simple branches. Often presents a beaded appearance due to spores present or irregular staining. The bacillus from bone or scrofulous tuberculosis is less virulent than that from other sources. They are more numerous in the active than in the more chronic processes. Microscopic examination of sections from old chronic lesions may be negative and culture or inoculation may be necessary to demonstrate their presence. ·

Modes of Infection.—*Inhalation.*—The lungs and respiratory tract are in a great majority of cases the primary seat of the tuberculous lesions. Tuberculous patients with advanced pulmonary changes expectorate countless millions of bacilli daily. When the expectoration is allowed to dry the virulent sputum in the form of dust is scattered far and wide. "The consumptive in himself is almost harmless and only becomes dangerous through bad habits" (Cornet). Infection by inhalation thus becomes the most frequent source of tuberculosis. The closer the contact with the patient the greater the danger, *i. e.*, in case of husband and wife, in families, in prisons, cloisters, barracks and hospitals. Nurses and attendants in hospitals for tuberculosis are not necessarily in as great danger as others owing to the better sanitation therein. The less the attention paid to prophylaxis, ventilation and hygiene the greater the danger of infection. *The expired air* of the consumptive is not infective but the moist *coughed* breath may be. Danger lies in handkerchiefs, beard, dusting, kissing, spitting, etc.

Milk and Meat.—Milk from tuberculous cows may contain the virus and thus communicate the disease to those who drink it. This danger is real and serious. The frequency of intestinal and mesenteric tuberculosis in children is thus explained. *Butter* may also convey it. The danger from eating tuberculous meat is rather remote though possible, the thorough cooking usually given, however, destroys the bacilli.

Inoculation.—Tuberculosis in man is rarely the result of inoculation and when so the resulting lesions are local. It sometimes occurs in those whose occupation leads to to the handling of dead bodies, dissecting room attendants, undertakers, butchers, tanners, or demonstrators of anatomy. Other sources of inoculation are circumcision, washing the clothes of tuberculous subjects, cuts from broken spit cups, the bite of tuberculous patients.

Hereditary transmission through a diseased mother, via blood through the placenta to the child. The great frequency of it in infancy and childhood and the localization of the lesions bears out this belief. Owing to the greater resistance of childhood the disease remains latent until the power of resistance is lowered by some other cause. Lymph glands, bones and joints are the usual site of the hereditary form. The pulmonary form is less common in infants and children. The possibility of infection in early life from tuberculous parents explains many cases supposed to be hereditary.

Conditions Favorable to Development. *Environment.*—Impure air, darkness, dampness, poor food, damp and poorly drained soil. *Individual Predisposition.*—Delicate constitutions, scrofulous diathesis, and in certain families the "tendency."

Age. None are exempt. It is most prone to attack those from eighteen to thirty-five years. *Sex.* Shows little influence, though females are slightly more prone to the disease owing to their sedentary, indoor life. *Race.* Negroes and Irish are the most susceptible. Hebrews are relatively immune. *Occupation.* Whatever causes crowding together in a dust laden atmosphere, as in mills, factories, or mines, predisposes. Glass and stone workers are especially liable. *Local Conditions.* Neglected catarrhs of the respiratory tract favor lower resistance, as do also the infectious diseases, measles, pertussis, etc., and chronic diseases of the heart, kidneys or liver. *Trauma.*—Injury may be an exciting cause—to the chest to the pulmonary, to the knee to the arthritic, to the head to the meningeal forms respecttively.

Evolution of the Tubercle.—The bacilli enter a given tissue or organs *via* of the blood, air or lymph current. They rapidly multiply and disseminate into the surrounding tissues with consequent irritation and the proliferation of connective tissue cells and the formation of epitheliod and giant cells with great increase of the leucocytes. The little induration thus formed constitutes the "tubercle." It degenerates in two ways: first, by Caseation. In the center the cells soften, lose their outline and the tubercle becomes a cheesy, homogeneous mass alive with bacilli. Second, by Sclerosis. After undergoing caseous degeneration, fibrous elements appear and multiply, usurping the place of the caseous matter until the tubercle becomes a dense hard nodular structure.

Diffuse Inflammatory Tubercle exists in the form of a diffuse, cheesy infiltration affecting various organs, such as the lungs, kidneys, liver, meninges, testes, spleen, etc. It is merely a "tubercle" on a large scale, the result of coalescence of many foci of inflammation with breaking down of the inter-cellular walls. It is rich in cell products and inflammatory exudate. If in the lungs the air vesicles of the involved area break down and become filled with these various products. The result is a caseous extensive tuberculous mass. In the lungs any sized area from a small lobule to a whole lung may thus be involved. Suppuration in tuberculous lesions is the result of a mixed infection by pus-organisms.

Miliary Tuberculosis. Acute General Tuberculosis.—So-called from "milium," the millet. Is an acute general tuberculosis, running a rapid course and characterized by the diffuse distribution of miliary tubercles in the various tissues and organs of the body. It is due to an auto-infection by the tubercular bacilli, caused by the presence somewhere in the body of a caseous focus, sometimes unsuspected but often ascertainable ; which ruptures into a vein or lymph vessel, more particularly the thoracic duct or the pulmonary veins. The bacilli are thus conveyed to the various tissues and a systemic infection running a rapid and malignant course ensues. The tissues most seriously affected are the lungs, pleuræ, peritoneum, cerebral meninges, lymph glands, spleen, liver and kidneys. The bacilli are unequally distributed to these different organs, hence the symptoms vary greatly according to which organ is most involved. Three forms are most distinctly recognized.

The General or Typhoid form in which the symptoms are those of a general infection resembling typhoid fever. The Pulmonary form in which the case strongly resembles a catarrhal pneumonia and the Meningeal variety or tubercular meningitis.

Added to these forms of tuberculosis we have the infection of the lymphatic glands of a chronic type commonly known as "scrofula."

PULMONARY TUBERCULOSIS.

Pulmonary phthisis, pulmonary consumption. Phthisis, from the Greek, meaning "to waste," popularly known as "consumption."

Tuberculosis of the lungs is the most frequent, fatal and interesting of the various forms of tuberculosis. It here presents a great variety of lesions; some characteristic, some of mixed quality, some belonging in common to other diseases, but *all marked by the presence of the bacillus tuberculosis.*

There are three forms of pulmonary tuberculosis. 1st. Acute pneumonic phthisis. 2d. Chronic phthisis. 3d. Fibroid phthisis.

ACUTE PNEUMONIC PHTHISIS.

Definition.—"Phthisis Florida," "Galloping Consumption." Is an acute pneumonic tuberculosis running a rapid course and presenting symptoms that in some cases resemble croupous pneumonia, in others broncho-pneumonia.

Symptoms.—The patient is seized with symptoms resembling pneumonia, chill or chilliness, fever, chest soreness or pains, cough, with expectoration, pulse rapid, respirations increased, areas of diminished resonance are discovered with dullness and bronchial breathing. In the *bronchial* form with various rales and scattered lobular consolidation; this is usual in children, especially after measles, and whooping cough. Or in the *croupous* form there may be rusty expectoration and consolidation of an entire lobe.

The patient may die in a few days from the intensity of the pneumonic process; may linger some weeks and die of exhaustion from hectic fever and general septic condition due to the local process, or at the end of four to six weeks may survive and apparently rally from the acute condition only to pass into a state of chronic phthisis.

Diagnosis.—Is very difficult at first; these cases so closely resembling pneumonia, and often go on to the time when a pneumonia would be expected to terminate without their tuberculous nature being suspected A case of pneumonia ushered in or accompanied by hæmoptysis is very suspicious. If by the twelfth or fourteenth day in a case of supposed pneumonia resolution or improvement does not take place, but, instead, the fever shows wide variations between the morning and evening records, there are periods of chilliness, with sweats evening or at night, the pulse is rapid and weak, the patient is much exhausted, anæmic, with no returning appetite, there is rapid emaciation, night cough; the expectoration muco-purulent and greenish in color, evidences of softening in spots previously dull, with many moist rales. All this should excite alarm and an examination of the sputum be made. If this reveals the presence of the tubercle bacilli the diagnosis of pneumonic tuberculosis may be conclusively made.

The broncho-pneumonic type is the most frequent, as acute tuberculosis is more prone to develop in children after measles or pertussis, those who are "run down," i. e., such persons as are predisposed to the catarrhal type of pneumonia.

CHRONIC PULMONARY TUBERCULOSIS.

Chronic phthisis; Chronic Ulcerative Tuberculosis of the Lungs.

Under this designation is found the large majority of cases, presenting the great variety of symptoms and lesions which make up the well known and familiar picture of chronic phthisis.

Morbid Anatomy.—The disease process first attacks the apices of the lungs and thence extends downward, probably by inhalation of the virus. The right apex is more frequently affected than the left. (Osler—in 427 autopsies found 172 in the right, 130 in the left, and 111 in both.) From the apex the disease extends to the apex of the lower lobe of the same lung and then attacks the apex of the opposite lung.

The primary lesion is usually from one to one and one-half inches below the extreme summit of the lung and this is equally true when it attacks the apex of the lobe below. Hence in physical examination the first evidence of the disease may usually be found in the supra-spinous fossa posteriorly, and just below the centre of the clavicle anteriorly. The primary lesion, when attacking the lower lobe, is first detected on the chest wall posteriorly at a spot opposite the *fifth* dorsal vertebræ. It is an axiom that "in a great majority of cases when the physical signs of disease at the apex are sufficiently definite to allow the diagnosis of phthisis to be made, the lower lobe is already affected." Hence, carefully examine this lower apex in suspicious cases.

It is interesting and important to remember that all the various processes and in every stage of development, may be found at one time in the same lung.

Lesions of Chronic Phthisis.—*Miliary Tubercles* are usually, but not invariably present. They develop in the alveolar walls or in the peri-vascular, peri-bronchial or sub-pleural connective tissue. They are found thickly grouped about the active lesions or distributed throughout the lungs.

Catarrhal or broncho pneumonia is most constantly present. Beginning in the terminal bronchioles it extends to the associated alveoli and both are soon filled with the products of inflammation in which the large flat aveolar epithelium predominate. In most cases there is a coincident pneumonic inflammation of the alveolar walls or frame work. These regions of inflammation and deposit constitute the

Areas of Consolidation.—These in a varying length of time undergo caseous degeneration. The process commencing at the centre of the area, gradually extending toward the periphery, encroaching more and more through the inflamed tissues. This central caseous mass ultimately softens, becomes purulent and there is found the

Cavity or Vomica.—The presence and pressure of the purulent contents favor further ulceration and necrosis and the cavity steadily increases in size, intervening tissues are destroyed and contiguous cavities unite until a lobe or even a whole lung may be honeycombed with small cavities, or the intra-alveolar frame work may break down entirely and form one large excavation. Those cavities communicating with a bronchus may thus empty themselves and their contents be expectorated or otherwise they remain filled with purulent matter. In the more acute and rapid processes there is no lining membrane and the walls are of ragged necrotic tissue. In chronic phthisis the walls are firmer and lined with a smooth, well-defined limiting membrane which constantly secretes pus. Even this does not prevent the gradual enlargement of the cavity by disintegration of adjacent lung tissue.

The bronchi and blood vessels resist the ulcerative process longest and they are frequently found exposed in these cavities. Blood vessels thus weakened by the destruction of thin supporting tissues, dilate and often rupture, thus causing frequent hæmorrhages, sometimes severe or even fatal.

Sclerosis.—May take place in a tubercular-pneumonic area that has been checked by treatment or favorable conditions before the stage of softening. This occurs by the development of fibrous tissue around the area, encapsulating it, or distributed throughout the mass. The slower the tuberculous process from restraint by medical,

hygienic or climatic treatment, the greater the tendency
and opportunity for healing by fibrosis.

Aside from the local processes above described there
are changes in other organs and tissues as follows :

The Pleura is almost always involved. Inflammation
may be simple, but is usually tubercular, showing adhesions of varying density and often with serous, purulent
or hæmorrhagic effusion and with miliary tubercle or
caseous masses in the thickened membrane.

The Bronchi are constantly affected with chronic catarrhal inflammation and the smaller tubes often show
bronchiectatic cavities.

The Bronchial Glands are inflamed, swollen, and show
caseous masses or purulent foci.

The Larynx is often involved and ulceration and distruction of the vocal chords and epiglottis is frequent.

Other Organs.—The brain, liver, spleen, kidneys, endo-
and peri-cardium and the intestinal tract are usually involved in secondary tuberculous processes. The latter
accounts for the troublesome diarrhœa often present late
in the disease.

Variations in Onset.—A typical case setting in with
fever, night sweats, cough, emaciation, anorexia, etc., is
usually soon recognized, but there are many cases commencing in an atypical manner; they may be thus classified:

Fever group, in which there is fever of intermittent, remittent or continuous-type with prostration and anorexia
—symptoms not distinctly pulmonary but suggesting
malarial infection.

Pleurisy group, with repeated attacks of pleurisy, usually the dry form but may be with effusion and retarded

recovery, gradually developing hectic symptoms pointing to the lungs.

Laryngeal group, showing huskiness, swelling, congestion and even ulceration of the laryngeal structures. These symptoms may be the first to excite suspicion but will be found secondary to established lesions in the apex of the lung.

Hæmoptysis group. In some cases a hæmorrhage is the first symptom to attract attention to the lungs, after which other pulmonary symptoms develop rapidly. Carefully examine and subsequently observe every case of hæmoptysis.

Bronchitis group, so often seen, so often overlooked until too late. A neglected or repeated "cold," receiving but little or irregular attention because seemingly of trifling import until a hæmorrhage, unusual loss of strength or weight, suddenly awakens to the true situation.

Symptoms.—These are divided for convenience of study into local and general.

Local Symptoms.—*Pain.* This may be present early and prove very distressing or may be absent altogether. It is usually due to the associated pleurisy and when so is some indication as to the locality of the lesions. There are often myalgic and neuralgic pains in various parts of the chest and soreness due to the strain of coughing.

Cough is almost universally present and remains throughout the course of the disease. At first it is dry and hacking, but later becomes hoarser and more paroxysmal with marked nocturnal aggravation. Laryngeal involvement gives a hoarse or husky quality to the voice or even aphonia. In a few cases cough is absent. By its nocturnal aggravation preventing sleep and its severity inducing vomiting of food, it becomes an important factor in increasing exhaustion and malnutrition.

Expectoration is quite constantly present. At first is catarrhal in character. When softening occurs, it becomes more free and muco-purulent in character. Later when cavities have formed it is profuse, greyish or greenish yellow and purulent. Sweetish in odor or fœtid from decomposition. Most profuse in the morning from the night's accumulation. It now assumes the so-called "nummular" form, *i. e.*, isolated flattened masses, greenish grey in color, airless and sinking when spat in water. The presence of greenish gray purulent masses in the sputum, with other suspicious symptoms, should warrant the making of a microscopical examination. If such reveals the presence of the tubercle bacilli the diagnosis of pulmonary tuberculosis may be conclusively made. If in addition elastic tissue is found, it indicates that degeneration and softening has taken place. *Blood* is not infrequently present in the expectoration. It may vary from a mere trace, tinging or streaking the sputum, to a severe hæmorrhage of clear blood. When present in minute quantities so that the sputum is only tinged or streaked with it, it is due to bronchial hyperæmia. When there is free expectoration of blood it comes from an eroded vessel. Copious or fatal hæmorrhage is due to the rupture of a dilated or weakened vessel exposed in a cavity.

Dyspnœa. Is not a marked feature unless there are pleuritic pains, large pleuritic effusion or rapid and extreme consolidation. The absence of it in these cases with their greatly diminished lung capacity is explained by the anæmia, or lack of corpuscular elements in the blood and the waste of tissue explains the lessened demand for oxygen.

Physical Examination.—It is well to remember that all signs may be present at one time in the same lung.

Inspection reveals "phthisical thorax," *i. e.*, unusual length, contraction, flatness and increased width of inter-costal spaces. Lack of expansion and unusual flatness of supra- and infra-clavicular regions with projection of scapulæ, like wings, behind.

Palpation. Increased vocal fremitus and lack of expansion, particularly of supra- and infra-clavicular region.

Percussion. Degree of impaired pulmonary resonance varies with the stage and extent of the disease process. A flat and high pitched note over the diseased area, especially in clavicular region anteriorly, the supra-spinous fossa and inter-scapular region posteriorly with the arms folded. Compare the diseased with the sound side. An area of consolidation centrally located and surrounded by normal or emphysematous tissue may seem resonant.

Auscultation. Voluntary increased force of respiration is often necessary to demonstrate clearly. Feebleness of respiration, impaired expansion over diseased area. Do not confuse with the general feebleness due to muscular weakness and debility from other causes. Prolonged expiration which is of higher pitch than inspiration and separated from it by an interval. Both are higher in pitch and harsher than on the normal side. "*Cog-wheel*" respiration consisting of localized interruption of inspiration, when associated with other signs, is of value and is most frequently heard in infra-clavicular region anteriorly.

Bronchial rales when localized and with localized pleuritic friction sounds when associated with other signs are strongly corroborative.

Cavities. The various signs thereof are best demonstrated with the patient's mouth open. They are shown by persistent bronchial breathing and absence of dulness over a limited area. Tympanitic percussion note over limited region surrounded by dulness is the most characteristic. "Cracked pot" sound is present when a cavity communicates with a bronchus. A well developed cavity shows bronchophony, amphoric breathing and gurgling rales. Percussion note of a cavity varies with the amount of superimposed dull or resonant tissue.

General Symptoms.—*Fever.*—A daily afternoon or evening rise of temperature without apparent cause should excite suspicion of phthisis. Fever is the most important symptom. It is usually remittent or intermittent and frequent observations should be made during the day. Incipient tuberculosis with fever of an intermittent type may be mistaken for malarial fever in regions where malaria abounds. The temperature curve shows great variation in different cases, but its usual form is an afternoon or evening rise reaching a maximum (102° to 105°) between two and six P. M., and a morning fall reaching a minimum between two and six A. M. In the early part of the disease the fever is of the remittent type, but with the breaking down and suppuration of lung tissue and the consequent systemic contamination the fever becomes more hectic in character, *i. e.*, intermittent. The morning hours will show a normal or subnormal temperature, but late in the forenoon there will be a gradual rise, reaching a maximum from 6 to 10

P. M. Chills or chilliness may usher in the fever at any stage of the disease, but are most constant after destructive changes have taken place. A continuous fever with a variation of not more than 1° occurring during the course of chronic phthisis is of serious import, indicating the presence of acute pneumonia.

Sweat.—Drenching sweats are a most common and distressing feature and may occur at any stage of chronic phthisis, but are most frequent and severe after cavities have formed. They usually follow the fever paroxysm and consequently appear during the night or early morning hours. Late in the disease a sweat may appear after sleep during any hour of the day.

The Pulse.—Is feeble, rapid, and easily compressible. This rapid, compressible and easily accelerated pulse is regarded as an early diagnostic sign of phthisis when associated with other suspicious symptoms.

Emaciation.—Progressive anæmia and loss of flesh is a characteristic and prominent symptom of chronic phthisis. Do not mistake the brilliant eye; scarlet lips and flushed cheeks of the hectic fever for health. The loss of weight is an indication as to the progress of the disease. An arrest of loss or a gain, is a favorable sign. The great emaciation of the later stages of phthisis is seldom equalled in any other disease.

Larynx.—Laryngitis is a very frequent complication and follows the pulmonary development of the disease. The various tissues of the larynx are inflamed, œdematous, ulcerate and may be destroyed by extensive necrosis. Huskiness of the voice is the first indication, followed by aphonia with intense pain upon speaking, coughing and swallowing. Important because of its serious effect upon nutrition.

Nervous System.—Variously affected, but the most serious complication is cerebro-spinal meningitis. The mind is usually clear throughout the disease in spite of months of fever, pain and exhaustion. The consumptive is proverbially hopeful. This is characteristic.

Pleura.—Pleuritis is usually present. It is most often the dry form, but may be purulent. Pneumo-thorax results from the rupture of a cavity into the pleural sac, leading to hydro- or pyo-pneumo-thorax.

Gastro-Intestinal Tract. — The buccal cavity often shows aphthous ulceration, and the soft palate, tongue, tonsils or pharyngeal walls may be the site of tuberculous ulceration. If associated with laryngeal ulceration these become serious factors by their interference with deglutition and nutrition. Anorexia is common, especially in the later stages. Nausea and vomiting are often present, due to reflex causes, gastric weakness or violent fits of coughing. Indigestion is frequent from various influences upon the stomach and its secretions. Diarrhœa, due to tuberculous ulceration of the ileum or colon, is a most distressing and exhausting complication, especially in the later stages of the disease.

Other Organs.—In protracted cases the terminal phalanges become clubbed and the nails markedly curved over their ends. The *skin*, especially over the chest, shows the stains of pityriasis versicolor. Œdema of the lower extremities is present late in the disease from cardiac weakness. *Endo-carditis, nephritis* and *femoral thrombosis* may occur as complications.

Diagnosis.—A careful and thorough physical examination, with a close investigation of the symptoms and clinical history, supplemented by a microscopical examination of the sputum, will establish the diagnosis. The early discovery of the disease is of the greatest importance to the patient and this fact emphasizes the necessity of thoroughness of examination in suspicious cases. The earliest signs are discoverable by auscultation of the apices where evidences of bronchial breathing and the rales of localized bronchitis are dangerously suggestive. The presence of elastic tissue in the sputum proves distruction of lung tissue.

Prognosis.—Many factors enter into the prognosis. In general it is unfavorable, though well defined cases may be cured as shown by the fibrous cicatricial tissue and evidences of former cavities found post-mortem. Some of these doubtless underwent the so-called " spontaneous cure," *i. e.*, without special treatment, and in some cases without the disease being suspected, nature by the formation of fibrous tissue isolated or filled the diseased area with scar tissue. Perfect recovery from well advanced pulmonary phthisis never occurs. The extent and stage of the lesions and especially the patient's persistence in treatment and ability to secure the benefit of proper diet, hygiene, climate and treatment all influence the prognosis. Tubercular meningitis, hæmoptysis and pneumo-thorax may bring on a fatal termination at any time. Laryngeal and gastro-intestinal complications are most unfavorable. Rapid emaciation and feeble digestion are especially unfavorable. In acute pneumonic phthisis the prognosis is always bad. The average duration of the disease is from two to three years.

Prophylaxis.—The danger of infection is practically only through the sputum. The latter should be caught in a proper receptacle and burned and not spat about upon the floor, street, or in handkerchiefs, where it may dry and be distributed and inhaled by others. The patient should sleep alone and the tuberculous should not marry. Infants and young children are most susceptible to infection. Hence a mother with tuberculosis should not suckle her infant and a child of tuberculous parents or of a family prone to phthisis should be most carefully watched and every attention given to its hygiene, diet, exercise, and minor ailments. Give special attention to the nose and throat and remove adenoids and hypertrophied tonsils. A family or the young persons in a family, so predisposed, should remove to a suitable climate before trouble develops. The milk and meat supply should be carefully inspected by skilled experts for the good of the whole community.

Treatment.—*General Measures.*—Nutrition controls the situation; as Osler aptly says, "make the patient grow fat and the local disease may be left to take care of itself." There are three indications in treatment. First, secure maximum degree of nutrition. Second, use such local and general measures as favorably influence the tubercular process. Third, alleviate symptoms.

Fresh Air.—Secure pure air, equable temperature and maximum amount of sunshine. A patient with a temperature of 100° or over should be at rest in bed. When the temperature remains below 100° the patient may take moderate exercise and gradually increase it with growing strength and endurance, but not to the point of fatigue or sufficient to cause a rise of temperature. Unless the weather is rainy or blustering the windows of the patient's room may be opened freely, avoiding a draught, or the patient, well protected, may sit, recline, or be carried on a cot to the veranda or lawn, and thus left exposed to the fresh air and sunshine for the greater part of the day.   Low atmospheric temperature nor the cough, fever, sweats or hæmoptysis do not contra-indicate this exposure to the air and sun, both of which inhibit and destroy the bacilli.   At night the sleeping room should be well ventilated.

Climate.—A patient with well developed cavities, hectic fever, sweats, and emaciation should not be sent from home.   The question of change of climate and where to send such patients is a matter for careful individualization and judgment. Briefly stated, cases with moderate, unilateral disease, limited to the apical region, and without much cavity formation or emaciation and in fair physical condition, do well, and stand a good chance of recovery from outdoor life anywhere, but especially in high or moderate altitudes, whether warm or cold, *i. e.*, Colorado, Arizona, New Mexico, Northern Maine and the mountains of Virginia or the Adirondack region.

In patients with bilateral disease and cavity formation there is little hope of permanent cure, and these do best in warm, low altitudes, *i. e.*, Southern California, Florida, South Carolina and Georgia (Aiken, Thomasville or Summerville).

Nervousness, emphysema, cardiac or kidney disease contra-indicate high altitudes.

Hygiene. — Phthisical patients should wear woolen underclothing, varying the weight to suit the season. They should, unless very feeble, resort to well directed exercise, carry the shoulders well thrown back and constantly think to take full, deep respirations and twice or thrice daily take breathing exercises. Warm bathing often enough to insure cleanliness and cold sponging of the throat and chest accompanied by deep breathing with friction and massage of the upper chest to aid in nutrition and expansion of the apices.

Diet.—This should receive special attention as it is most important. Each case must be studied as to personal idiosyncrasies and the digestive power and the diet varied or modified to suit the situation. Generally speaking, a liberal meal of the various articles of food is most suitable at the usual meal hours, while between meals and at bedtime a portion of some liquid or concentrated nourishment should be given, *i. e.*, milk, egg in milk, koumyss, broth, gruel, grapes or grape juice or one of the various predigested foods. Cream, butter, fat meat and oil are of value when they can be taken and are tolerated by the stomach. Malt beverages may whet the appetite and increase weight.

The stomach must be catered to and when it is weak or there are intestinal complications the diet must be modified to suit the individual case.

Stimulation. —Judgment should be used in the employment of stimulants. The routine administration of alcoholics is of no particular benefit. A little good red wine with meals may aid digestion and improve nutrition. Port, sherry or tokay wine may be taken alone or with an egg between meals. The indications for the stronger alcoholics are in the later stages when there is great prostration, weak heart, anorexia, emaciation and general feebleness. They are particularly required in the early morning hours during the period of subnormal temperature and exhaustion following the sweat. Whiskey or brandy, two to eight drachms, with water or in a milk-punch or eggnog.

Remedial Treatment.—Various drugs, methods and serums have been advocated as possible specifics from time to time, particularly during the last few years. They have received the attention of the profession under circumstances to give them a thorough trial. While each of these has been found to possess virtue with limitations, not one of them has demonstrated sufficient specific action in tuberculosis to warrant its being depended upon as the soverign remedy in this distressing malady. The best treatment resolves itself into careful prescribing for the symptoms or special conditions as they arise, coupled with the best, dietetic and hygienic measures.

For the special symptoms the following remedies are variously indicated, the relative demand for their use seeming to be in the order mentioned:

Pre-Tubercular State.—General hectic condition, ill-defined and suspicious, but without well marked physical signs calls for *Bacillinum* or *Tuberculinum.*

The Totality of a case of tuberculosis seems most often covered by *Phosphorus, Arsenicum iod., Stannum iod., Ferrum phos., Ferrum ars., Iodine, Antimonium iod., Kali carb., Chininum ars.*

Fever.—*Baptisia, Ferrum phos., Arsenicum iod., Chininum ars. Aconite* is contra-indicated because of the liability to contract cold after its use.

Cough.—*Stannum iod., Antimonium iod., Phosphorus, Sanguinaria, Rumex crisp.* Heroin $\frac{1}{12}$ to $\frac{1}{20}$ grain or Codeine $\frac{1}{4}$ to $\frac{1}{12}$ grain, in tablet or vehicle, may be used as a palliative if necessary.

Sweat.—Dilute Phosphoric acid, ten to twenty drops in four ounces of water and taken in divided doses during the day, is excellent. *Cinchona, Ferrum ars., Pilocarpine* 2x. *Agaricine* 1x, one grain at bedtime. Atropine, $\frac{1}{200}$ grain hypodermatically at bedtime. A cup of weak chamomile tea drank upon retiring is often very efficacious as is also a cool sponge bath with water acidulated with vinegar.

Hæmoptysis.—*Millifolium, Hamamelis, Geranium mac.*, the latter in mother tincture, five drop doses. Absolute rest, cold liquid food, ice cap to the chest, heat to the feet. See chapter pulmonary hæmorrhage.

Pain.—If pleuritic, *Bryonia alba., Aconite, Kali carb., Squilla.* Exposure to the arc light is valuable to relieve the pain of the pleurisy. If myalgic—*Bryonia alb., Actea rac.*, or Acetanalid five grains as a palliative. Paint the painful region with tincture of iodine or employ massage.

Laryngeal Inflammation. — *Causticum, Phosphorus, Drosera, Iodine, Spongia, Arsenicum iod.*

Intestinal Tract.—Papoid one to three grains or pepsin three to five grains, alone or with Bismuth subnitrate five to ten grains, taken after eating is excellent in indigestion or diarrhœa. A good pleasant formula is ℞. Bismuth subnitrate ʒiv, Essence of pepsin ʒvi. Mix. S. Take one dessertspoonful after eating. Burned brandy one or two drachms frequently repeated is of value. Opiates are contra-indicated. Persistent diarrhœa due to intestinal ulceration is benefited by colon flushing with hot boric acid or carbolized water or weak flaxseed tea. Of the remedies to be used are *Cuprum ars., Cinchona, Ferrum ars., Veratrum album.*

Special Suggestions.—*Cod liver oil* given in one drachm doses after each meal is excellent in its effect upon nutrition.   It acts best in children and especially in bone and glandular tuberculosis.   Gastric irritability or fever contra-indicate its use.   A dessertspoonful of emulsion of mixed fats or thick cream is a good substitute.

Strychnine nitrate or sulphate $\frac{1}{80}$ to $\frac{1}{100}$ of a grain three times daily aids digestion and gives nerve and cardiac strength.

Ichthyol combined with glycerin in equal parts and given two drops after each meal, increasing one drop per dose daily, until twenty to thirty drops are given at a dose, gives good results in cavity cases but not when associated with enteric troubles.

Creosote or Guaiacol have been favorites for their effect in diminishing the cough and expectoration.   They are given in one drop doses after eating and gradually increasing to eight or ten drops.   ·

Inhalations of Guaiacol, Terebene, Creosote Benzoin, Iodine or Eucalyptus, one drachm to the pint of boiling water, are sometimes useful as antiseptics to the respiratory tract and sooth the cough.

Sunlight.—The patient stripped to the waist and exposed to the direct rays of the sun in a warm room will be benefited as to the cough, sweats, fever and local pains, but this should not be tried if there is much exhaustion.

Electricity.—The ozone inhalations from static electricity are claimed to stimulate and improve nutrition.   The X-ray is of value as a diagnostic means.   The X-ray and high frequency currents are as yet too much in their infancy to draw definite conclusion as to their action in tuberculosis. They have benefited many cases, apparently by improving nutrition and general cell tone, thus inhibiting the disease. Upon the bacilli their effect is to cause rapid growth and over-development with great increase in numbers, leading to ultimate attenuation and extinction from overstimulation.

FIBROID PHTHISIS.

Definition. — Chronic Interstitial Pneumonia. Cirrhosis of the Lung. Consists in a gradual fibroid change in which fibroid tissue takes the place of normal or tuberculous lung tissue, with consequent contraction and induration.

Etiology.—Most cases supervene upon an arrested tuberculous process, though some are of simple pneumonic nature. In the cases of tuberculous origin, the fibroid change is more common in the apex, where it surrounds the cavity formed or invades areas of caseous degeneration, arresting the active process and producing shrinkage and hardening, changing the area, lobe or lung into a mass of tough, grayish, fibrous tissue. This retraction leaves the bronchi dilated and inelastic, forming bronchiectatic sacs.

Fibrous phthisis of non-tubercular origin may be the method of termination in unresolving lobar or bronchopneumonia. In the first the walls of the alveoli and the fibrinous deposit filling them undergo fibroid change. In the catarrhal pneumonia the finer bronchi, the alveoli and their contents are affected by the fibrosis and the lobules become hard fibrous masses, with no trace of normal lung tissue left. Fibroid change in the lung may take place after attacks of plastic pleurisy with extensive adhesions and resulting lung compression.

Symptoms.—This disease is essentially chronic, lasting ten to twenty years, during which the patient may enjoy a fair degree of health. The patient is usually thin, anæmic and suffers dyspnœa upon slight exertion, but with little or no serious constitutional disturbance, *i. e.*, fever sweat, etc. There is much cough with purulent expectoration, sometimes fœtid, from the existing bronchiectasis.

Physical Signs.—These are characteristic. The chest on the affected side is sunken, flat, retracted and immobile. The shoulder is drawn down and the spine bowed. When the right lung is affected the heart may be drawn by the retraction toward the affected side; when the left lung is the seat of trouble, the area of cardiac impulse is greatly increased. Percussion shows variation from flatness over apex or base, to amphoric or tympanic resonance over bronchiectic cavities. Auscultation gives cavernous breathing sounds at the upper part and feeble sounds mixed with rales at the base.

Treatment.—Is only for intercurrent affections or aggravation of the cough. The primary condition is not amenable to treatment. The patient should seek a mild climate and avoid exposure to inclement weather. The remedies and means of service are those usually required for chronic bronchitis, bronchiectasis and emphysema.

BRONCHO-PNEUMONIA.

Definition.—Known also as acute catarrhal pneumonia and lobular pneumonia.

Broncho-pneumonia is a catarrhal inflammation attacking the air cells in various lobules of the lungs. It is usually bilateral and is the result of an extension from a bronchitis of the smaller tubes and is therefore secondary in character.

Etiology.—This form of pneumonia is due to an invasion of the air cells by continuity of surface, obstruction of the bronchioles or inhalation of irritating secretion, of an inflammation previously existing in the bronchial tubes. It may supervene in some cases in atelectatic lung tissue and in some rare instances the same irritating influence that causes the bronchitis may excite the catarrhal pneumonia spontaneously. Age is a most important factor, a great majority of cases occurring in infancy and old age, particularly when the constitution is debilitated or enfeebled. It is especially liable to occur by extension during the course of the various infectious diseases, whooping cough, measles, influenza, diphtheria and variola. Bad hygiene, improper nourishment, in fact, any debilitating influence are potent predisposing causes. The inhalation of irritating substances, vapors, and various kinds of dust frequently excite an attack.

Pathology.—The morbid changes are confined to various groups of air cells (lobules) scattered throughout the lungs. These may be here and there or several that lie close together may be involved, thus giving a larger area of consolidation and simulating pneumonic fever (croupous pneumonia) by the seeming involvement of a whole lobe. These consolidated areas appear as nodules varying in size from that of a pea to a hazelnut scattered throughout the affected lungs. They may lie near the surface of the lung in which case they appear as small round elevations, or may be more deeply seated through the tissue. They do not fill when the lung is inflated, they are not as tough as healthy lung tissue and break down easily upon pressure, they vary in color from red to bluish or they may in some instances be firm, dry and whitish as if they had undergone purulent infiltration. When cut these nodules exude a reddish fluid or a few drops of dark blood. The lung tissue surrounding the inflamed nodule will be found to be congested, œdematous or emphysematous. In broncho-pneumonia we recognize three stages to the pathological process, though these are not as well defined as in lobar pneumonia. The *first stage* is one of vascular engorgement, the alveolar epithelium is swollen and turgescent, with more or less desquamation and exudation. The air cells are filled with serous fluid rich in cellular elements, blood and epithelium. The *second stage* is that of complete consolidation. The air cells are full of exudate rich in pus cells, blood cells and desquamated epithelium. The *third stage* is the time when this deposit undergoes fatty degeneration and softening and is absorbed or expectorated, with a subsequent restoration of healthy epithelium. In unfavorable cases the deposit undergoes cheesy or purulent degeneration leading to gangrene, abscesses, interstitial pneumonia or becomes infected with the bacilli of tuberculosis. Atelectasis frequently results from the broncho-pneumonia of children and localized pleurisy is not uncommon when the inflamed lobules lie near the surface of the lung.

Symptoms.—The earlier symptoms are essentially those of the accompanying bronchitis of the smaller bronchial tubes. It is sometimes very difficult to determine just when lung tissue becomes involved. But when in the course of a bronchitis, whether simple or associated with some other disease, there is a gradual rise of temperature to 103° or 105° (but not the chill and sharp rise of fever seen in lobar pneumonia), respiration becomes difficult and increases in frequency to 50 or 80 per minute, with the complaint of soreness and pain ; the pulse grows rapid (140—160), loses force and is compressible; the soft, loose cough of the preceding bronchitis becomes dry, tight and hard with pain and deep soreness; expectoration is slight or absent—if present it is muco-purulent or blood streaked (not " rusty " as in lobar pneumonia), then the invasion of a lobular pneumonia may be diagnosed. Fatal cases are due to the respiratory condition and symptoms. The respirations become frequent, labored, feeble and short, the extraordinary muscles of respiration with the alæ nasi are brought into play, the heart systole grows weaker with feeble pulse, clammy extremities and cyanosis, death occurring from heart failure due to respiratory failure. In favorable cases the temperature lowers, respiration becomes deeper and less frequent and labored, the cough loosens, expectoration becomes freer and the pulse grows stronger. In the chronic form the pulse and respiration gradually increase in frequency, the temperature is never as high as in the acute, rarely going above 102°. There is dyspnœa, loss of appetite, strength and flesh and a general systemic failure. Death in such cases occurs from general exhaustion and cardiac failure, not from respiratory failure as in the acute form.

Physical Signs.—Percussion shows isolated points of consolidation, vocal fremitus being increased over these areas. Auscultation shows fine mucous rales over the affected areas, heard during inspiration and expiration and of a metallic character, indicating pulmonary consolidation.

Complications and Sequelæ.—Bronchitis is present in all cases. Pleurisy in many cases is a complication, accounting for the respiratory pain, especially if the lobules involved are near the surface of the lung or the area of inflammation is extensive. Intestinal catarrh is a common complication in children and infants and is a serious factor. Convulsions may occur and are of grave import; in fact, the brain symptoms in severe cases may resemble those of meningitis.

Diagnosis.—The diagnosis of a lobular pneumonia, supervening as it does upon an existing diseased condition, is often difficult, especially in mild cases with a limited invasion. The inflammation being limited to small and scattered areas of lung tissue surrounded by healthy lung tissue renders the detection of consolidation most difficult. Thus one of the most reliable signs of the disease is not available, and for the same reason bronchial or broncho-vesicular breathing is not marked. The physical signs are those of bronchitis with the added evidence of limited localized areas of consolidation. The crepitant rale is a reliable sign, but is naturally masked in these cases by the moist rales of the co-existing bronchitis of the finer tubes. From croupous or lobar pneumonia, catarrhal pneumonia is distinguished by its bilateral and scattered development, the gradual onset, supervening upon another preceding disease, its lobular and not lobar character, and in adults by the mode of invasion. From a rapid tuberculosis which it often resembles, the bacilli should be looked for, their presence or absence deciding the diagnosis.

Capillary bronchitis and catarrhal pneumonia so nearly resemble each other clinically that some recent writers and teachers do not treat of them separately. The clinical diagnosis between them is usually well-nigh impossible. In simple capillary bronchitis the temperature runs a lower course as a rule, the prostration is more marked, defective aeration is very pronounced and we fail to find any areas of consolidation. Capillary bronchitis, like catarrhal pneumonia, is the result of an extension into the finer bronchioles of the inflammation starting in the larger tubes, but unlike catarrhal pneumonia there are not areas of consolidation nor the general aggravation of all the fever symptoms that mark the development of the latter.

Prognosis.—In infancy, during old age or cases in which the patient is in an enfeebled condition the outlook is not favorable. The prognosis is affected by coexisting circumstances. Bad nutrition, unhygienic surroundings, rachitic children, chronic nephritis or cardiac complications render it unfavorable. The probable outcome is less encouraging when the pneumonia complicates whooping cough, than when associated with measles. The height of the temperature, the extent of the bronchitis and the amount of consolidation are most important factors. A temperature of 104° to 105° is unfavorable. The ultimate prognosis in cases not going on to

complete resolution is unfavorable, as such areas of consolidation form foci for tubercular infection or abscesses.

General Treatment.—As broncho-pneumonia occurs
in systems already depleted by previous disease, the
tendency is to exhaustion, hence the indications are to
build up the general nutrition and strength, accompanied
by remedies to overcome the acute inflammatory process.
The patient should be kept at rest in bed; his position
should, however, be very frequently changed. Light or
liquid nourishment in concentrated form should be frequently administered. Evidence of impending heart
failure should be promptly met by the administration of
alcoholic stimulants or Strychnine in one-hundreth grain
doses. Respiratory failure takes place from obstruction
of the air vesicles and finer bronchioles, hence to combat
this, employ friction and massage of the respiratory muscles and, when possible, respiratory exercises, deep breathing at intervals, several times daily, artificial respiration,
or, best of all, the use of oxygen (as described under
pneumonic fever). Emetics are of little value, as the depression resulting from their use more than overbalances
the relief they afford. Alternating hot and cold water
douches may be necessary in infants threatening suffocation. During the important and critical period of convalescence the patient should receive most careful attention to avoid relapse and to ensure complete recovery.
Respiratory exercises, diet, exercise, clothing, hygiene,
etc., should be carefully supervised. Cod liver oil,
mixed fats, malt preparations, fresh air and change of
scene with appropriate remedies constitute the treatment
for this stage.

Remedies.—*Aconite.*—Chill or chilliness, sudden rise

of fever with thirst, restlessness and shifting pains. Cough is short, dry and hacking. General aggravation of all symptoms indicating that some new development is taking place. For the first hours of invasion.

Antimonium arsenite.—Valuable in broncho-pneumonia of the aged, with the loose rales and threatened suffocation of antimony associated with the thirst, restlessness and feverish prostration of arsenic.

Antimonium tartaricum.—The most frequently indicated remedy in broncho-pneumonia. Loose cough, chest full of mucus with fine rattling rales. Patient is too prostrated to raise the accumulated secretion which threatens to suffocate. Face pale or cyanotic and covered with clammy sweat, extremities cold, pulse quick and feeble, respiration rapid and oppressed, the whole ensemble one of distress and threatened suffocation.

Bryonia alba.—Cough dry, hard and deep-seated, breathing is oppressed, with soreness and sticking pains, indicating pleuritic involvement, some scanty mucous expectoration, with rawness and pain during coughing effort.

Ferrum phosphoricum.—Anæmic cases with asthenia. Less fever, thirst and restlessness than *Aconite*, but more debility. Hard, dry cough with oppression and expectoration of blood-streaked mucus. Not of use after cyanosis appears.

Iodine.—High fever, hard, croupy cough, marked areas of consolidation, strumous subjects. Valuable in stage of hepatization. Give in low potencies.

ipecac.—Bronchial tract filled with mucus, loud rattling rales. Loose suffocative cough, with nausea, gagging or vomiting.

8

Lachesis.—Low condition. The cough is spasmodic and suffocative, waking suddenly from sleep and easily excited by touching the throat or laryngeal region. Difficult respiration, constantly obliged to take a deep breath. Threatened paralysis of the lungs with cyanosis and great distress for breath, especially after sleep. Extreme prostration.

Laurocerasus.—Dry cough or with copious expectoration. Cyanotic condition with great constriction of the chest, gasping for breath, small, feeble pulse, threatened paralysis of the lungs.

Lycopodium.—Cough, with grey, salty expectoration. Dyspnœa, with sense of constriction, shortness of breath and intense weakness. Great difficulty to breathe, with fan-like motion of the alæ nasi. Aggravation from four to seven each afternoon.

Opium.—Cough, with dyspnœa and blue face. Apathy, to a heavy stupor. Difficult, rattling, intermittent respiration, with hot, sweaty skin and drowsinesss and coma.

Phosphorus.—Especially suitable to the hectic type of fever and patient. Much oppression of breathing, with tightness across the chest. Hacking cough, with moderate expectoration of blood-stained mucus.

Squilla.—Chest shows much rattling of mucus which is expelled after violent coughing. The latter causes sharp sticking pains and is accompanied by involuntary micturition. Eyes suffused and watery, thin nasal discharge with excoriated nostrils. This remedy has the loose cough of *Antimonium tartrate*, but without its prostration, while the pains are like *Bryonia*, but the coryza and free secretion are different.

Sulphur.—May be used with advantage in protracted cases as an intercurrent. Also follows well after other remedies during the period of convalescence to promote resolution and absorption of secretion with return to the healthy state.

Veratrum album.—Deep, hollow cough, with much expectoration, suffocation, blueness of the face, weakness, with coldness of the surface and extremities and cold, clammy sweat on the forehead. Collapse and threatened heart failure.

ATELECTASIS.

Definition.—Atelectasis is a condition in which the walls of the pulmonary alveoli are collapsed. It may be divided, as to origin, into the congenital or acquired, and as to form, into the diffuse or lobular. In fœtal life atelectasis is the normal condition of the lungs and its persistence after birth constitutes the congenital form.

Etiology—*Congenital* atelectasis is due to lack of pulmonary development or power to expand the lungs. This may arise from the general feebleness found in children born prematurely; or an early separation of the placenta, compression of the cord or a protracted labor, may cause the child to make breathing efforts before it comes into the world, thus drawing liquor amnii or mucus into and obstructing the bronchioles.

Secondary atelectatsis or the *acquired* form is the most usual and generally is the result of bronchial obstruction, due to plugs of mucus entering the smaller bronchioles during an attack of bronchitis and permanently closing them; the air in the terminal air cells beyond the point of obstruction is gradually absorbed and the cell walls collapse. This is especially apt to occur in the bronchitis secondary to measles or whooping cough, owing to the enfeebled condition of the inspiratory muscles. Patients enfeebled by rachitic or wasting diseases or bad hygiene are particularly liable to pulmonary collapse during a course of bronchitis. The pressure upon a bronchial tube of an aneurism, an enlarged gland or intra-thoraric tumor may cause collapse.

Pathology.—The lobules affected are depressed below the surface of the lung; they are darker than normal in color and do not crepitate. When cut they appear dense and tough. The lower and posterior portion of the lungs are most affected in the congenital form, while in the acquired the collapsed lobules are diffused throughout the lung tissue. The microscope shows the alveoli completely collapsed containing only a little secretion.

Physical Signs.—In the congenital form, atelectasis may be readily recognized, if it is well marked, by a distinct retraction and inactivity of the chest wall over the inferior ribs posteriorly, due to lack of expansion. In these cases percussion shows dulness, but in the acquired form such areas may be so small and so scattered throughout the lung tissue as not to be discoverable by percussion. Auscultation reveals the rales of the associated bronchitis only, but if large areas are involved in the collapse there may be an absence of respiratory sounds.

Symptoms.—In the congenital form the symptoms are more or less severe according to the extent of the area involved. Fever is absent and the symptoms are those of obstructed respiration. Rapid breathing with cyanosis, cold extremities, feeble pulse, etc. In the acquired form, if during an attack of bronchitis the breathing becomes suddenly more rapid and difficult with developing cyanosis and depression of temperature with evidence of exhausting vitality, atelectasis may be diagnosed if the physical signs corroborate the symptoms. It is most apt to be confused with lobular pneumonia, and if the areas collapsed are small and scattered a clear diagnosis may be impossible as it usually is associated with lobular pneumonia. In the congenital form, if a new-born infant makes rapid, feeble efforts to breathe, is short of breath when nursing, and has a blue skin and feeble cry, *without rales or cough* (and the heart sounds are normal) atelectasis may be diagnosed.

Prognosis.—Is bad if an extensive area is collapsed. It is stated that one-fourth the mortality of early infancy is due to this condition. The outlook in the acquired form following measles and whooping cough is particularly grave.

General Treatment.—In the congenital form respiratory efforts should be encouraged by slapping, sudden application of cold, artificial respiration, etc. Crying should be encouraged. The physician may apply his mouth to the child's and distend its lungs with air from his own, holding the infant's nose while he does so. An emetic may be given if the bronchial tubes seem filled with mucus with inability to expectorate. Drugs are of little use in this form. In the acquired form of atelectasis, attend to the underlying diseased condition, nourish and build up the patient as rapidly as possible. To stimulate deeper respiration and thus aid in expansion of the collapsed alveoli, instruct in deep breathing, employ massage, use cold douching, passive gymnastics or electricity. All these are helpful. In event of threatened suffocation inhalation of oxygen should be employed.

Remedies. –The remedies should be those for the associated condition:

Antimonium arsenite.—Restlessness, thirst, fever, sweat and perspiration. Great dyspnœa, threatening suffocation with cyanosis and fine rales.

Antimonium tartaricum.—Is particularly well indicated with its excessive mucous accumulation, rattlin grales, inability to expectorate, cyanosis and exhaustion.

Carbo vegetabilis.—Great oppression, wheezing and rattling in chest, extreme collapse, with bluish color and coldness of the breath and body surfaces.

Lachesis.—Short oppressed breathing with suffocative attacks, ropy mucous expectoration with great dyspnœa. Threatened paralysis of respiration, especially when waking from sleep.

Lycopodium. — Emaciation with bloated abdomen. Atony and apathy. Cachectic children, cough, dyspnœa, labored effort to breathe with motion of alæ nasi. Relief from warm food and drink and 4 to 8 P. M. aggravation.

Sambucus.—Suffocative cough with presence of much mucus. Child turns blue and gasps for breath. Worse just after midnight.

EMPHYSEMA.

Definition.—Emphysema is over-distension of the air vesicles accompanied by loss of elasticity and power to contract, with ultimate atrophy of the alveolar walls, resulting in permanent dilatation of the aveoli.

Varieties.—There are several varieties.

Compensatory.—Whenever one lung or a part of one lung is prevented by disease from fulfilling its functions the neighboring healthy tissue or the opposite lung takes up the double work and the vesicles become distended from the extra effort. This is the case with broncho-pneumonia, tuberculous areas, pleural adhesions, cirrhosis of the lung or pleurisy with effusion.

Vesicular.—The acute distension from bronchitis of the finer tubes with threatened cyanosis, in cardiac asthma, angina pectoris, or pressure on the pneumogastric nerve; the violent efforts to get air in any of these may result in sudden distension and even rupture of the air cell walls.

Interstitial. — During violent coughing, straining at stool or after tracheotomy, air may appear in the inter-lobular or subplural tissue.

Atrophic.—Senile changes involving atrophy of the alveolar walls with distension of the vesicles. Most frequently seen in withered up old people.

Hypertrophic.—This is the usual variety, characterized by enlargement of the lungs due to distention of the air cells and atrophy and relaxation of their walls, with resulting dyspnœa and evidence of imperfect æration of blood.

Etiology.—Emphysema results from persistent high intra-vesicular pressure acting upon congenitally weak lung tissue. Due to defective nutrition in the alveolar structure and deficiency in development of the elastic fibres. Heredity plays as usual an important part. As exciting causes may be mentioned anything which induces forced inspiration or expiration. Asthma and chronic bronchitis are the most frequent causes, whooping cough, violent prolonged exertion, players on wind instruments, glass blowers, etc.

Pathology.—The thorax becomes capacious, barrel-shaped, and the cartilages are calcified. The lungs are large and have lost their elasticity. The air vesicles are much distended, many are coalesced, producing greatly enlarged cells with atrophy of the frame work and absence of elastic fibres. In the bronchi the mucous membrane is rough, thickened, and the finer bronchial tubes are much distended.

Symptoms.—Dyspnœa is constant or is produced by slight exertion. Respiration harsh, wheezy and much prolonged. Cyanosis is present in varying degree, sometimes very marked, even startling, and out of all proportion to the patient's apparent comfort and ability to get about. This feature is characteristic, for the same degree of cyanosis if due to heart disease or other variety of lung trouble would mean that the patient would be in bed and near death. Bronchitis with cough is a constant symptom, with relief in summer and aggravation in winter. Asthma is frequently present. As age increases recurrent attacks of bronchitis occur and the condition grows worse. Death occurs from intercurrent pneumonia, cardiac dropsy, or cardiac distension and cyanosis.

Physical Signs.—Inspection shows the chest to be barrel-shaped, the antero-posterior diameter being equal to the lateral. The sternum and costal cartilages are prominent, the inter-costal spaces are widened, with immobility during respiration.

Palpation. The apex beat is rarely felt, but there is pulsation in the epigastrium. Percussion gives greatly increased resonance, full and drum-like. Heart dulness

obliterated and liver line of dulness lowered. Auscultation gives breathing sounds enfeebled with a prolonged
expiration (4–1 instead of 1–4) harsh and rough, accompanied by coarse rales.

General Treatment —Emphysema is incurable as far
as correcting the morbid changes already established in the
air vesicles; the process, however, may be arrested.
Establish a sound digestion and give a rich nitrogenous
diet, avoiding starch and sugar. Alcohol and tobacco
are injurious and should be forbidden. A milk diet,
peptonized or with lime water, may be necessary in those
of perverted or feeble digestion. Protect the patient
from cold and dampness. Outdoor exercise is beneficial,
avoiding, however, everything that will increase respiratory effort. The cough must be kept in check by
appropriate remedies aided by mild palliatives if necessary. Inhalation of oxygen will give much relief in
severe cases with marked cyanosis.

Remedies.—There are no remedies for emphysema
per se.

*Antimonium arsenite, Antimonium tartaricum, Kali
bichromicum* and *Ipecac* are most frequently indicated for
the associated chronic bronchitis. Also *Calcarea carbonica* for fleshy females who perspire easily and with
copious menstruation. *Calcarea phosphoricum* for old
men with atheromatous blood vessels. *Lycopodium* in
flatulent dyspeptics with excess of uric acid and gouty
symptoms. *Antimonium arsenite, Grindelia robusta,
Ipecac* or *Lobelia inflata* for the frequently accompanying asthma. Gastric symptoms call for *Argentum nitri-
cum, Lycopodium, Carbo vegetabilis* or *Nux vomica*. In
the later stages with cardiac weakness *Arsenicum album*
2x, *Strychnia nitrate* 2x, or *Digitalis* θ may be required.

PULMONARY HYPERÆMIA.

Definition.—Pulmonary hyperæmia consists in an engorgement and over-distension of the pulmonary vessels with blood. It is found in two forms, the active and passive, which will be described separately.

Active Hyperæmia.—This form is a sudden engorgement of the lungs with blood, not an independent disease, but rather a condition, similar to the first stage of various inflammatory diseases of these organs, but terminating before the actual inflammation is established.

Etiology.—Among the causes may be mentioned cold, chilling the body surface suddenly, inhalation of irritating gases or substances, embolic obstruction to the flow of blood through the capillaries, the result of violent heart action from over-exertion or excitement. Alcoholism is a predisposing cause.

Pathology.—The vessels of the lungs and mucous membrane lining the bronchi are distended with blood, with resulting high color. Some œdema is present with a flow of blood-stained frothy serum into the vesicles.

Symptoms.—There may or may not be a chill, followed by some fever. There is always, however, a severe degree of dyspnœa and oppression, stitching pains, cough with frothy, rust stained expectoration, even bloody or amounting to actual hæmoptysis. Physical examination shows feebleness of respiratory sounds, approaching to bronchial breathing, the resonance is impaired, with subcrepitant rales.

Diagnosis.—Is based on the sudden onset with determining cause, great dyspnœa and an absence of the signs of other acute pulmonary disease. Resembles pulmonary œdema, but the associated cardiac or renal disease differentiates the latter, though often separation is difficult as each is usually accompanied in some degree by the other.

Prognosis.—Is usually favorable, unless leading to pneumonia. Some fatal cases are reported after violent exertion or exposure to cold.

General Treatment.—Rest in bed, heat to the feet, mustard or flaxseed poultices applied to the chest with the use of hot foot baths.

Remedies.—*Aconite.*—Sudden violent attack from exposure or chilling the body surface. High fever, thirst, restlessness, great anxiety. Shortness of breath, oppression, with stitching pain and hot feeling in the lungs. Dry, hacking cough. A leading remedy.

Bryonia alba.—Fever, thirst, tightness and oppression across chest, with hard, dry, racking cough, and sticking pains, aggravated by motion and cough.

Ferrum phosphoricum.—Anæmic, debilitated persons. Hard, dry cough with sore chest and expectoration of blood-streaked mucus or pure blood. Best remedy for delicate subjects.

Phosphorus.—Hard, dry, racking cough from tickling in the throat pit. Tightness across the chest with a sense of great weight and oppression. Respiration rapid and labored with feeling of heat in the lungs. Voice hoarse and expectoration rusty or blood-streaked. The most popular remedy.

Veratrum viride.—Violent congestion in full-blooded persons. Thirst, nausea, high fever, with throbbing, bounding pulse and red face, Difficult breathing with sensation of a heavy load on the chest.

Passive Hyperæmia.—This variety of pulmonary congestion occurs in two forms, the hypostatic and the obstructive.

Hypostatic Congestion—Hypostatic Pneumonia. —This occurs at the base of the lungs and is due to the combined effects of a weak heart, blood changes, relaxed blood-vessel walls and gravity. Met with in protracted diseases where the patient is exhausted and lies much upon the back. Particularly prone to develop in the aged and enfeebled. Often occurs in profound nervous diseases, tumors of the brain, apoplexy, traumatic affections, opium or carbonic acid poisoning, and after surgical operations.

Pathology.—The changes are to be found in the bases of the lungs posteriorly, which are engorged with blood and serum, the alveoli filled with corpuscles and epithelial cells. This portion of the lungs becomes deep bluish red. The condition is due to gravitation of blood to the most dependent portions. At times it amounts to actual hepatization, the so-called hypostatic pneumonia. Œdema is usually present to some extent.

Symptoms.—These are not well marked; they are discovered by careful physical examination based upon the favoring conditions. Cyanosis in varying degree may be present, with extreme prostration. There is evidence of consolidation, especially in the base of the lung on the side usually lain upon, with feeble breathing, bronchial in character, and fine, moist rales. Frequent examinations should be made in all conditions favoring pulmonary stasis.

Prognosis.—Is always unfavorable because of the gravity of the primary condition. Hypostatic congestion is an evidence of profound exhaustion and cardiac weakness and must be promptly met, as it is an indication of the utmost gravity.

General Treatment.—Change the position of the patient very frequently. Give the most nourishing and easily assimilated diet. Rectal enemata of nourishment may be necessary. Employ stimulation to meet the cardiac weakness and relieve circulatory stasis. Bathing with alcohol accompanied by massage is beneficial. Strychnia nitrate in $\frac{1}{50}$ to $\frac{1}{100}$ grain doses will often tide over a crisis with its tonic effect on the heart.

Remedies.—The remedies are those indicated for the underlying diseased condition, but this complication may suggest such drugs as *Ammonium carb.*, *Antimonium tart.*, *Arsenicum alb.*, *Baptisia*, *Carbo veg.*, *Digitalis*, *Muriatic acid*, *Phosphorus* and *Rhus tox.*

Obstructive Congestion.—This form is due to the mechanical influence of various diseased conditions in the left heart or to the presence of new growths, in preventing the free flow of blood through the pulmonary vessels.

Pathology.—The lungs become distended with blood; they are consequently larger, heavier and firmer. The connective tissue hypertrophies and the coats of the blood vessels thicken. Hæmorrhages into the connective tissue takes place, producing pigmented spots, with forcing of blood cells into the air vesicles tinging the sputum. The lungs from lack of oxidation take on a dark brown color. This state is known as "Brown Induration."

Symptoms.—Are those of the existing heart disease, palpitation, oppression, cough, dyspnœa, all aggravated

by exertion. Hæmoptysis is not uncommon and the
sputum is often tinged with blood; feeble pulse, inspiratory rales, oppression, etc., with existence of heart disease, establishes the diagnosis.

Diagnosis.—If in case of heart disease the patient
complains of cough, dyspnœa, spits blood and crepitant
rales are discovered; the diagnosis of this form of pulmonary complication is simple.

Prognosis.—A chronic condition of obstructive congestion of the lungs may maintain for years, its gravity
depending upon the cardiac condition. Aggravation of
the pulmonary symptoms (great dyspnœa, hæmorhages,
etc.); especially with cyanosis, is of grave import, indicating a rapid cardiac failure.

Treatment.—Is that of the co-existing heart lesion.

PULMONARY HÆMORRHAGE.

Definition.—Pulmonary hæmorrhage occurs in two
forms: 1st. Broncho-pulmonary hæmorrhage, in which
the blood is expelled into the bronchial tract and is duly
expectorated. 2d. Pulmonary apoplexy or pulmonary
infarction, in which the blood escapes into the air cells
and areolar tissue of the lungs themselves.

**Broncho-pulmonary Hæmorrhage or Hæmop-
tysis.**—Etiology.—In this form the exudation of blood
is due to a variety of conditions: 1st. It occurs sometimes in young people of either sex; the hæmorrhage
will be quite free, but no cause discoverable. No evidence of pulmonary disease and no effect upon the general health. 2d. In connection with diseases of the

lungs, tuberculosis, pneumonia, cancer, gangrene, abscess and bronchiectasis or in ulcerative conditions of the larynx, trachea or bronchi. 3d. As a result of certain heart affections, notably, mitral lesions and in aneurisms, in which case the blood may ooze through the sac or the latter may rupture. 4th. In females in the form of vicarious menstruation. In malignant diseases with blood degeneration (typhus, typhoid, purpura hæmorrhagica, etc.). And at times in the gouty diathesis.

Symptoms.—Hæmoptysis usually comes on suddenly. The patient experiences nausea, and a warm, sweetish, salty taste in the mouth as it fills with blood; there is a cough and blood is expelled. It may be only a few drams and the trouble ceases or there may be the expectoration of small quantities for several days at a time. If, however, an aneurism has ruptured or a large blood vessel given way the flow of blood will be profuse, the patient will struggle to expectorate it, signs of asphyxiation will appear and life flicker out, literally drowned. Fatal hæmorrhage may occur into a large phthisical cavity without external manifestations of blood. The blood in hæmoptysis is light in color, frothy, mixed with mucus, of alkaline reaction, and the clot contains air cells.

During and for some time subsequent to an attack of hæmoptysis auscultation will reveal the affected chest-region filled with profuse rattling rales. The mucous expectoration may be blood-tinged for days after an attack of hæmoptysis. The patient usually has some indication of an approaching hæmorrhage, a sense of constriction and uneasiness during inspiration that he cannot account for. During the hæmorrhage the countenance looks pale and anxious, he becomes tremulous and often faints; this is not due so much to the amount of blood lost as to the mental shock at the knowledge that a pulmonary hæmorrhage is taking place. The pulse is rapid and tense and the temperature subnormal, though it may temporarily rise to 103° just afterward. When the temperature rises to 102° or 104° after a hæmorrhage and remains so it indicates that the attack was the initial symptom of an acute tubercular pneumonia. There is greater prostration from a pulmonary hæmorrhage than from any other loss of blood in like quantity.

Diagnosis.—The physician has to diagnose hæmoptysis from hæmatemesis. The patient can usually tell whether the blood was coughed up or vomited. The blood from the stomach is dark in color, clotted, mixed with the ingesta, partaking of the latter's odor and with acid reaction. Its expulsion was accompanied with nausea and vomiting. It should be borne in mind that blood from the lungs may gush out rapidly, be swallowed and subsequently vomited, but in that case nausea and vomiting follow the hæmorrhage. Each case should be carefully investigated, if obscure, to ascertain that the blood does not come from the nose, naso-pharynx or gums, and that the patient is not malingering.

Prognosis.—It is well to remember that the *immediate* effects of an attack of pulmonary hæmorrhage are usually recovered from in spite of the seemingly alarming prostration, pallor and syncope that attend it. Excepting, of course, such cases as are due to the rupture of a large blood vessel or aneurism. The *ultimate* outlook, however, is unfavorable, as in the majority of cases pulmonary hæmorrhage is associated with some serious, though perhaps unsuspected, disease or is the precursor of pulmonary phthisis, acute or chronic.

Pulmonary Infarction.—**Etiology.**—Known also as Pulmonary Apoplexy, is that condition in which the bleeding takes place into the air cells and interstitial tissue of the lungs. The hæmorrhage, as a rule, is limited, and is caused by the blocking of a branch of the pulmonary artery by a thrombus or embolus. This condition is most frequently met with in chronic heart disease.

Pathology.—Infarctions usually occur at the surface of the lung and are in the form of a pyramid with the base toward the periphery; the pleura over this area is usually inflamed. An infarction appears like a blood clot, dark and firm in texture, but as time goes on it becomes red or brown. They vary in size from that of a walnut to an orange, according to the degree of the bleeding. The artery leading to the infarction will be found stopped by thrombus or embolus, and if the blood vessel be a large one the hæmorrhage may occupy a whole lobe. In some instances a stoppage of a large branch of the pulmonary artery will not result in the formation of an infarction, owing to the bronchial blood vessels and the extensive ramifying capillaries being able to carry on the circulation. The outcome of an infarction is variable. In some cases it is doubtless re-absorbed and the circulation resumed. In others, if the patient lives, the clot undergoes the usual changes and remains permanently as a shrunken, dense, fibrous mass. Sloughing, abscess, or gangrene may result.

Symptoms.—The manifestations of pulmonary infarction are obscure. It may be suspected when hæmoptysis occurs in association with chronic heart disease, particularly mitral regurgitation. If the hæmorrhage is extensive there may be symptoms of loss of blood with

9

shortness of breath and evidence of consolidation over the site of the infarct.

General Treatment.—The prime indications in the treatment of pulmonary hæmorrhage are to reduce the frequency of the heart beat and to lower blood pressure. As the most important aid in attaining this, perfect repose of body and peace of mind should be secured and rigidly insisted upon. The patient should lie down in a comfortable position, preferably on one side, to favor the easier expectoration of the accumulated blood. The diet should be light and unstimulating. Alcoholics are contra-indicated. Water increases blood pressure and should only be taken in small quantities. Ice may be sucked freely. The temperature of the room should be low, but the extremities kept warm with hot bottles. The patient should be encouraged to expectorate with as little effort as possible and the cough which is present held in check (voluntarily or by formulas given in the treatment of acute bronchitis). The patient is mentally depressed and despairs from the first, hence should be strongly reassured. In the management of these cases they may be divided into two classes: 1st. Those cases of moderate bleeding due to the transudation from highly engorged blood vessels or congested mucosa, with possible capillary rupture. 2d. Those violent and often fatal cases which are due to the rupture of a large blood vessel or aneurism. In the first classification, where the bleeding takes place in a moderate degree, the indicated drug (see Remedies) with the general measures suggested will prove all-sufficient and satisfactory. If, however, the bleeding is profuse and persistent the situation resolves itself into an alarming mechanical problem in which the indicated remedy should be promptly supplemented by active styptic measures lest the patient's life-current ebbs away without his having received the benefit of all known means of relief. In these severe cases ice bags or ice water compresses should be applied over the bleeding area, which may be located by the rales. The application of ice should not be resorted to unless necessary and should be discontinued as soon as the hæmorrhage is controlled, owing to the danger of broncho-pneumonia following hæmorrhages when ice has been used. Free catharsis with saline laxatives (Magnesium sulphate ʒiv) lowers blood pressure and is indicated in plethoric individuals. Ligating the extremities sufficiently to prevent venous return also lowers the pressure in the pulmonary vessels. The cough in ordinary cases is a necessary aid, as it is desirable to get the accumulated blood out of the bronchial tubes, but if constant and harassing it will increase the bleeding and should be checked by Morphia sulphate, ⅛ to ¼ grain, hypodermatically. This composes the patient, lowers blood pressure, stops the cough and thus materially aids in controlling the hæmorrhage. The fluid extract of Ergot, one drachm every two to four hours or one drachm in four ounces of water, and given one teaspoonful every one-half to one hour. This is an old and well-tested favorite when the amount of blood expectorated is considerable.

Ergotole may be used hypodermatically in doses of twenty or thirty drops every three or four hours.

Among the newer remedies that has already stood severe testing in the field of hæmorrhage—pulmonary and otherwise—and seems to promise a brilliant future, is Adrenalin chloride, Solution 1–1000. Five drops every half to one hour until relieved and continued three times daily for ten days.

In persistent moderate hæmorrhage the powdered supra-renal gland in three grain tablets or capsules, given one three times daily after meals, is of benefit.

Remedies.—*Aconite.*—High arterial tension, bounding pulse, flushed face, anxiety, nervous excitement, hacking cough, with bright frothy expectoration.

Arnica montana.—Bleeding of dark clotted blood, with soreness and pain. After injury or overexertion.

Cinchona.—An excellent remedy to give after hæmorrhage to relieve the pallor, ringing in the ears, faintness, etc. These symptoms in some cases are more due to fright than to the amount lost.

Digitalis.—May be called for in the mother tincture after severe or repeated hæmorrhage, for the prostration, feeble pulse and cold extremities.

Ferrum phosphoricum.—Frequent slight hæmorrhages, frothy blood-tinged mucus, with cough, tightness and oppression. Particularly in anæmic persons or phthisical subjects.

Hamamelis Virginica.—The cardinal remedy for passive, painless bleeding, showing venous characteristics. In tincture or distilled extract.

Hydrastinine hydrochlorate is strongly endorsed by Dr. Wm. C. Goodno for pulmonary hæmorrhage. He advises its use in the second decimal trituration or in urgent cases in ¼ grain doses hypodermatically.

Ipecac.—Active, bright red bleeding, with severe cough and loose bubbling rales, especially with cold sweat and nausea.

Millefolium.—One of the best remedies. Easy flow of bright blood, with cough, oppression of the chest and palpitation. Given in the tincture.

PNEUMONOKONIOSIS.

Definition.—A fibrosis of the lung tissue, due to the inhalation of dust in various occupations. The condition has received several special names according to kind of dust inhaled: Anthracosis, from coal dust; Chalicosis, from lime and stone dust; Siderosis, from mineral dust, iron, etc.; Byosinosis, from cotton and ordinary dust; Tabacosis, from tobacco dust.

Etiology.—Dust in various forms is always present to a certain degree in the air we breathe. In the ordinary quantity it is doubtful if it ever reaches the air vesicles, as it is caught by the naso-pharynx and the mucous membrane lining the bronchial tubes, thence it is swept into the larger bronchi and expectorated. When, however, dust is present persistently and in large quantities these forces are inadequate and the dust particles lodge in the finer bronchioles and air cells, penetrating the deeper structures and producing morbid changes. Workers in dusty occupations are short lived. The average age of grindstone makers is only twenty-four years. In coal mining districts the death rate from lung disease is very high.

Pathology.—The lungs become enlarged and increased in weight. There is a chronic bronchitis and bronchiectasis, with much thickening of the walls. The bronchial glands enlarge and connective tissue increases in the interlobular septa, resulting in inelasticity and emphysema. The pleura becomes thickened.

Symptoms.—Are those of bronchitis, bronchiectasis and emphysema, with muco-purulent expectoration containing the particles or stains of the inhaled dust.

Treatment.—Is that of the diseased conditions mentioned. Change of occupation is imperative, with abundance of fresh air, and all possible measures to improve the general health.

PULMONARY CARCINOMA.

Definition.—Cancer of the lung may be primary or secondary, but is usually the latter, and all varieties are found.

Etiology.—The cause is the same as of cancer elsewhere. This development, however, is not common. It may occur at any age except in the very young. Heredity is an important causative factor. Usually develops as secondary to cancer of the breast, but may follow cancer in any other part. Takes its origin in the epithelial and glandular structure of the bronchial mucous membrane.

Pathology.—In frequency, the variety most usual is the medullary or encephaloid, scirrhus less often, epithelioma or melanotic very rarely. The disease usually develops as nodular tumors, multiple in character and appearing in several places at once. By coalescence a large tumor is formed involving a good portion of a lobe. The bronchial glands become enlarged, the pleura is studded with nodules, pleurisy develops and effusion usually takes place. Death, as a rule, occurs before extensive pulmonary involvement takes place, but if the patient survives the cancerous nodules soften, ulcerate, break down, and cavities form.

Symptoms.—There are none especially characteristic of pulmonary cancer per se. Cough, expectoration and pain varying in intensity and location are usually present. So, if in the course of cancer elsewhere, these symptoms appear with evidence of localized consolidation, rales and pleurisy, the diagnosis may safely be made. If the cancerous tumor attain considerable size it may produce difficult deglutition, dyspnœa, aphonia, pulmonary hæmorrhage or œdema, by pressure upon the œsophagus, trachea, recurrent laryngeal nerve, or branches of the pulmonary veins, respectively.

Prognosis.—Malignant disease in this location is invariably fatal, its duration depending upon the general state and vitality.

Treatment.—Look to the diet and general care of patient. Remedies as suggested for cancer elsewhere and special medicine to relieve urgent symptoms as they arise.

PULMONARY GANGRENE.

Definition.—Necrosis and death of lung tissue. May be circumscribed or diffuse.

Etiology.—Entrance of the bacteria of putrefaction into portions of the lung tissue already degenerated by inflammatory stasis or suppuration. Underlying such a termination must be a predisposition of constitutional mal-nutrition and vital depression. Poorly nourished, half-fed, illy-clothed wrecks of humanity and those who are exposed to all the vicissitudes of weather are particularly liable, especially if they are the victims of Bright's disease, diabetes or habitual intemperance. In such persons pneumonia, bronchiectasis and tuberculosis with cavities offer the larger quota of instances.

Pulmonary embolism frequently is a cause of **gangrene**, either by cutting off the nutrition to a part or by carrying infection to the tissues from bed-sores, puerperal septic inflammations or suppurating caries. Another cause is the decomposition of food inhaled by the insane, idiots, or in cases of paralysis of the muscles of deglutition.

Typhus, variola, measles, glanders, pyæmia and septicæmia and animal venoms may result in gangrene.

Pathology —The lower lobes are most often affected. It may be a circumscribed area, from the size of a chestnut to a butternut, or small spots may be found scattered through the whole lung. Occasionally the entire lung may be replaced by a putrid gangrenous cavity. The affected tissue may be brownish, greenish or black, and firm or containing sanious fluid. A line of demarcation may form and the necrotic tissue soften and be expelled. The bronchial tubes are the last tissues to be affected.

Symptoms.—These vary with preceding pulmonary lesion. Sudden and great asthenia, not in proportion to the physical signs, elevation of temperature, often to a high point, and very offensive sputum suggest the presence of gangrene, where the local condition and the constitutional state are favorable. The sputum is usually thin, sanious, green, brown or black and horribly offensive. Chills, sweating, vomiting and diarrhœa accompany as well as the usual symptoms of pulmonary trouble—cough, dyspnœa, etc. There are evidences of consolidation or cavities with bronchial rales.

Diagnosis.—The characteristic, indescribable fœtor of the sputum, with consolidation and excavation, the rapid course (" fœtid bronchitis " is slow and not violent), the profound cachexia, with the underlying condition and history of the case, establishes the diagnosis.

Prognosis.—Is always unfavorable. Invariably fatal in the diffuse form and rarely a recovery in the circumscribed cases. Usually fatal within a week of the initial chill. Death is due to exhaustion, hæmorrhage, or following a peritonitis, pleurisy or pneumo-thorax, due to perforation.

General Treatment.—Should be directed to the patient's strength until the necrotic tissue is cast off. Rich, highly nutritious dietary, eggs, milk and broths, with stimulation. Sprays by inhalation to secure antisepsis of the cavities affected, carbolic acid, iodine, creosote or thymol. Incision of the cavity with drainage is to be considered if the necrosis is localized.

Remedies.—*Arsenicum album.* — Great exhaustion, restlessness, nightly aggravation, mental anguish, thirst, high fever, burning pains, vomiting, dark offensive diarrhœa, dyspnœa and thoracic distress, all make this a remedy which is often most suitable.

Echinacea.—With its foul discharges, low septic symptoms, chilliness, nausea and depression. It is a remedy particularly suitable to septic, malignant and gangrenous affections. Give 5 to 10 drops of the tincture every two hours.

Lachesis.—Blood decomposition, low septic state, system profoundly poisoned, great prostration, throat sensitive, cyanosis, skin bluish or purplish, worse after sleep, relief after offensive expectoration.

PULMONARY ABSCESS.

Etiology.—Abscess of the lung may arise from a variety of causes. 1st. Those following local inflammation of various kinds in the lungs themselves. Wounds, operations, suppurative conditions, etc., in the respiratory tract above the lungs, the infective matter may be inhaled, causing local suppuration. 2d. Embolic, abscess from infective embolisms which are carried into the lung vessels from a purulent condition elsewhere. 3d. Traumatic, from perforating wounds, foreign bodies, or a perforating abscess of the liver. 4th Those suppurations occurring during the course of tuberculosis.

Symptoms.—When in the course of any disease likely to cause pulmonary abscess local symptoms of the lung appear, or those already present become aggravated, with cough, impeded respiration, higher fever, rigors, profuse sweats, great prostration, purulent expectoration, etc., especially if a localized consolidation, followed by cavity, can be determined, with discharge of a large amount of pus, the diagnosis is reasonably certain.

Diagnosis.—Abscess may be differentiated from gangrene by the horrible fœtor and necrotic tissue of the latter. From empyema by the previous history of pleurisy and the greater amount of pus. From hepatic abscess by the pus of the latter showing bile and being brownish in color.

Prognosis.—Is always grave, though may recover if carefully nursed and treated. In hepatic or pleuritic abscess discharging through this channel the prognosis is bad.

General Treatment.—Build up and sustain the patient's strength to withstand a long period of suppuration. Give a highly nutritious diet with stimulation. Drainage may be possible.

Remedies.—*Arsenicum iod.*, *China off.*, *Hepar sulph.*, *Lachesis*, *Silicea*, are most frequently indicated.

PULMONARY SYPHILIS.

Etiology.—Is a rare affection. Due to general syphilitic infection, either hereditary or acquired, and occurs as follows:

1st. *White pneumonia* of the fœtus, in which in the fœtus or new-born the lung is firm, heavy and airless, with greatly indurated alveolar walls. The color is whitish gray, the so-called "white hepatization."

2d. *Gummata* from the size of a pea to a goose egg may be scattered throughout the lung.

3d. *Fibrous pneumonia* beginning at the root of the lung and extending along the bronchi, with gummata. Is limited to this area.

Symptoms and Diagnosis. — The former are not characteristic and the latter is most difficult. The symptoms are usually those of bronchiectasis or chronic interstitial pneumonia. In those cases suffering from syphilis in general, with obscure pulmonary symptoms of fibrosis or bronchiectasis and no bacilli are in the sputum, syphilis may be assumed.

Treatment.—Consists of the same measures and remedies as are indicated for the management of syphilis elsewhere.

PULMONARY ECHINOCOCCUS.

Definition.—Cysts are found in the pleura and lungs by the development of the tænia echinococcus. This is a small worm of three or four segments and a head having four sucking surfaces and a roseola of hooklets. Their development causes the formation of large numbers of multiple cysts containing fluid. Commonly called Hydatids.

Symptoms.—If small, their presence, either in the lungs or pleura, causes few symptoms, but as they grow and multiply, symptoms of compression, inflammation, cavities connecting with the bronchi and expectoration of fluid containing the hooklets. During life, unless the hooklets are found, it is usually diagnosed as phthisis or gangrene.

Treatment.—Is strictly surgical. Open and drain if possible. Injections into the sac are also used.

IV.

Diseases of the Pleura.

IV.

DISEASES OF THE PLEURA.

PLEURITIS.

Definition.—Pleuritis, commonly known as pleurisy, is an inflammation of the pleura, limited or general. Divided, according to duration, into the acute and chronic; according to form, into the plastic (dry or adhesive) and pleurisy with effusion.

Etiology.—Pleurisy may occur primarily as the result of exposure or traumatism, or secondarily in association with various diseases, pneumonia, tuberculosis and all other diseases of the lungs, or with the various infectious diseases, also with Bright's disease and rheumatism. The tuberculous origin of many pleurisies has been demonstrated.

DRY, PLASTIC OR ADHESIVE PLEURISY.

This form is usually localized. The attack begins with chilliness, moderate fever; sharp, sticking pain in the affected region, more when breathing, and a short, dry cough which causes pain. Friction sound is distinctly heard over the inflamed area during respiration and is due to the rubbing of the dry and roughened pleural surfaces together. It is this friction that causes the pain.

After a few days, under appropriate remedies and hot
applications, the symptoms disappear. During the
height of the inflammation a thin, fibrinous, exudative
layer forms, and this aids in the formation of the adhesions between the roughened pleural surfaces, which are
so common after a "dry" pleurisy.

PLEURISY WITH EFFUSION—SERO-FIBRINOUS PLEURISY.

Definition.—That form of pleurisy in which there is a
large accumulation of serous exudation.

Pathology.—Many cases of this form are microbic in
origin, especially tuberculous. The exudate is thin,
light, straw color and translucent. In some cases the
effusion takes on a bloody character, particularly in infectious fevers, cirrhosis of the liver, cancer and Bright's
disease. This form is known as hæmorrhagic pleurisy.
In other cases bands of adhesion form, dividing the effusion into various pockets. This is termed encysted pleurisy. In sero-fibrinous pleurisy the inflammation is more
generally distributed than in the dry or plastic form.

Symptoms.—The attack begins with a chill or chilliness, followed by a rise of temperature to 102° or 103°,
rarely more. There is a short, dry, hacking cough;
sharp, lancinating pain, aggravated by breathing, coughing or motion, and usually located in the infra-maxillary
region. Dyspnœa is present, at first due to pain, but
later to compression of the lung by the effusion. The
patient lies on the back or painful side. The fever lasts
from one to four weeks and may disappear before the ex-

udate does. As the fluid forms the pain decreases, but the oppression of breathing gradually increases in proportion to the rapidity and amount of the effusion forming. It is well to remember that cases may come on insidiously and the patient attend business until the dyspnœa, feebleness and emaciation demand attention. As the disease progresses there is constipation, anorexia, feebleness and emaciation.

Physical Signs.—*Inspection* shows impaired motion of the affected side, which appears enlarged, with filling out or obliteration of the intercostal spaces. *Palpation.* Vocal fremitus is diminished and the heart impulse is displaced according to the side affected and the amount of effusion. *Percussion* shows dulness beginning at the base of the lung posteriorly and extending up to a line corresponding to the level of the effusion. The dulness varies in degree according to the amount of fluid, amounting in cases of large accumulation to flatness, excepting at the upper portion of the lung, and that is dull. The opposite lung is often hyper-resonant. There may be some dulness after absorption takes place because of the thickened membranes and failure of the long-compressed lung to expand. *Auscultation* reveals friction sound until effusion takes place, when it disappears. Vesicular breathing grows more and more feeble as the fluid accumulates, and finally disappears, its place being taken by bronchial breathing.

Diagnosis.—The symptoms and physical signs are usually sufficient to determine the diagnosis. If doubt exists, a sterile hypodermic needle may be inserted in the fifth or sixth interspace on a line with the center of the axilla, or posteriorly on the same level. The sudden

10

violent onset, severe chill, high fever, rusty sputum and
the disturbed pulse-respiration ratio distinguishes lobar
pneumonia.   Whether the pleuritis is tuberculous or not
is determined by the history, obstinacy, emaciation and
hectic fever.

Prognosis.—Is usually favorable, except it be tuberculous in nature; may, however, be protracted in course
and adhesions are usually left.

PURULENT PLEURITIS—EMPYEMA.

Etiology.—Purulent pleuritis may occur primarily,
i. e., purulent from the start.   This is more frequent in
children and not usual in healthy individuals; or, as a
sequence of serous-fibrinous pleurisy, this again is not
usual in healthy individuals.   The secondary pleurisies
occurring as complications or sequelæ of the various infectious diseases are usually purulent in character, notably in scarlet fever, typhoid and many tuberculous cases.
Purulent pleurisy may result from local causes, fracture
of a rib, penetrating wounds, malignant diseases of the
lungs or œsophagus, and perforation of tubercular cavities
into the pleuritic cavity.   Microscopically the fluid in
empyema has the characteristics of ordinary pus.   It
may be fœtid in some cases, especially after perforating
wounds or in cancer or gangrene of the lung.

Physical Signs.—Practically are those of serous pleurisy, except that the greater weight of the fluid causes
more bulging of the lower intercostal spaces and greater
displacement of the heart or liver.

Symptoms.—Empyema may come on insidiously with

few chest symptoms, especially if during other diseases . or following sero-fibrinous pleurisy. But the symptoms of septic infection are generally present, anorexia, pallor, weakness, sweats and irregular fever. A cough in this form is not always constant.

Other Varieties.—*Tuberculous*, with the symptoms of sero-fibrinous or purulent pleurisy. *Hæmorrhagic pleurisy* or *hæmothorax*, occurring in the pleurisy of asthenic states, cancer, chronic nephritis, tuberculosis and the malignant fevers. *Interlobular pleurisy*, involving the serous surfaces between the lobes. *Encysted pleurisy*, in areas isolated by bands of adhesion. *Chronic pleurisy* occurs in two forms: First, chronic pleurisy with effusion, coming on insidiously or following the acute form, the fluid remaining in a variable quantity for years unchanged. Second, chronic dry pleurisy (*a*) as a sequence of ordinary pleurisy with effusion, the membrane thickened, dense, adhesive, some limitation of lung expansion and variable pains. (*b*) Following plastic pleurisy, the "primitive dry pleurisy," with thickening and adhesions.

General Treatment.—The patient should be kept at rest in bed and fed a light, nutritious diet. In the early stages flaxseed poultices or hot fomentations are beneficial and give grateful relief from the pain. In severe cases an excellent method is to strap the affected side during expiration with overlapping strips of adhesive plaster three inches wide. They should reach from the spine to the sternum. Codeine or Morphine in one-fourth to one-twelfth grain doses may be deemed necessary at intervals during the period of agonizing pain, but other means usually suffice. In the stage of effusion a dry diet, limiting the quantity of liquid taken to eight or twelve ounces daily, will check and reduce the amount of effusion.   A more active step in robust patients is to combine the dry diet with a dose of Sulphate of Magnesia (four to eight drachms) administered each or every other morning.

Thoracentesis should be resorted to when the rapidity of the exudation produces severe dyspnœa, feeble pulse, cyanosis, etc., or in protracted cases where, in three weeks, the fever having subsided, the patient is exhausted, with no decrease in the amount of the fluid.   The operation is not a serious one, but should be done under all antiseptic precautions.   A few drops of Cocaine solution, five per cent., may be previously injected at the site of puncture to ease pain, and the skin may be slightly incised, if the needle used be a large one, to facilitate its introduction. The patient's arm should be brought forward and the hand placed on the opposite shoulder.   The aspirator needle should be introduced close to the upper border of the rib (to avoid wounding the intercostal artery) in the sixth or seventh intercostal space in the mid-axillary line. The fluid should be withdrawn slowly and the amount should depend upon the amount of effusion and the length of time in forming.   More in proportion may be withdrawn from a rapid effusion than one more slowly formed.   Stimulants should be at hand, and severe pain, dyspnœa, cyanosis, violent cough or faintness, should call for their use and a cessation of the operation.   This operation is not only palliative, but curative, in many cases, even if only a portion of the fluid be removed.   It is a proceeding seldom demanded in children unless the case is purulent.   It may have to be repeated in the aged. Purulent collections in children will sometimes disappear by absorption without drainage.

Remedies.—*Aconite.*—Indicated in the early stage. Chill or chilliness, fever, thirst, restlessness, dry cough and sharp pains.

Bryonia alba is the classic remedy for the dry or plastic pleurisy, but becomes of less value as the fluid increases. The patient has sharp lancinating pains in the affected region, worse from motion or coughing. The cough is dry, hard or hacking, but restrained because of the pain. The patient lies on the painful side, breathing is repressed, there is fever, thirst, headache, furred tongue and constipation.

Ferrum phosphoricum for dry pleuritis in hectic or phthisical persons.

Kali carbonicum.—Prostration, cough, with tough expectoration; sticking pains with early morning aggravation.

Squilla.—Dyspnœa, with stitching pain in left side; short, rattling cough. For a dry pleurisy with a loose cough.

Sulphur.—Short, dry cough, with thoracic stitches and soreness, worse from motion. To complete the cure.

These remedies are usually sufficient to relieve a simple dry pleuritis. In those cases going on to sero-fibrinous exudation, as the fluid forms the acute symptoms of fever, pain, etc., gradually diminish and another variety of symptoms appear calling for another class of remedies.

Apis mellifica.—General tendency to serous exudation and dropsies. Valuable to promote absorption.

Arsenicum album.—Often indicated for the prostration, emaciation, dyspnœa, restlessness, fever, thirst, etc.

Arnica Montana is useful in pleurisy of traumatic origin or otherwise, with the characteristic sore, lame, bruised sensation and pain. Bed feels too hard. Pleuro-dynia.

Cantharis.—The most valuable remedy to promote ab-sorption in the exudative stage. Rawness and burning, with burning pains Vesical tenesmus. Acts best in the tincture, five to ten drops in four ounces of water, and one teaspoonful given every two hours.

Colchicum or *Rhus toxicodendron* in cases of rheumatic disposition or history, especially from exposure to raw winds or from getting wet.

Sulphur.—Is most valuable to promote absorption of fluid in cases that reach a standstill. May be used inter-currently with other remedies.

Purulent pleurisy is usually not considered amenable to remedies except in children, but in them and in some others much may be accomplished by the use of carefully selected drugs especially is this true after operation, which consists of resection of a portion of one rib, and thorough drainage, with frequent washing out of the cavity.

Silicea, Sulphur, Calcarea carb., Hepar sulph. and *Ar-senicum iod.* are of particular value in these cases to aid in the cure.

HYDRO-THORAX.

Definition. — Hydro-thorax is a non-inflammatory pleuritic effusion of thin, serous character and is a part of the general dropsy resulting in cases of chronic heart disease, in which case it is usually unilateral and on the right side. It also occurs in kidney disease, anæmia and other conditions, such as malaria, profuse diarrhœa, etc., inducing great blood impoverishment; these latter cases are bilateral.

Physical Signs are those common to pleurisy with effusion.

Symptoms are those of the associated disease plus dyspnœa, orthopnœa, cyanosis. There is no pain and no fever. Expectoration, if present, is thin, frothy and watery.

Treatment.—Aspiration should be performed if necessary, but postpone it as long as possible owing to the tendency to recur. (See "Thoracentesis" in pleurisy with effusion.) The use of saline purges may temporarily reduce the amount of effusion.

Remedies.—*Arsenicum album.*—Oppression of breathing with ascites and anasarca; scanty, frothy expectoration. Rapid, weak pulse; pallor, emaciation, restlessness and anxiety, thirst, faintness, anæmia and exhaustion.

Apocynum cannabinum.—Nausea, vomiting, drowsiness, difficult breathing, thirst and gastric irritability, with scanty urine and general evidence of dropsy. Acts best in appreciable doses. The tincture, ten drops three or four times daily, or better still, an infusion, one teaspoonful every four hours, gradually increased.

Digitalis.—Irregular, difficult breathing, with sighing; weak, intermittent pulse, with faintness; œdematous swellings, with scanty urination. Particularly in cardiac disease. Give the infusion, one teaspoonful every three or four hours, and increase. The tincture may be used in five to fifteen drop doses in a like interval.

Sulphur.—As a supplemental remedy in long-lasting

and obstinate cases, where the urgent symptoms subside and some effusion is left. To promote reaction and absorption.

PNEUMO-THORAX.

Definition.— The entrance of air into the pleural cavity. This accident is most frequent in male adults and is usually rapidly followed by pleural inflammation and effusion, which results in hydro-pneumo-thorax or pyo-pneumo-thorax.

Etiology.—This condition arises from a variety of causes, the most common being the rupture of a tuberculous focus or cavity during the course of pulmonary phthisis, less frequently by the perforation of the pleural sac by abscess, gangrene or malignant disease either of the lungs or adjacent organs. Wounds and injuries to the chest or the strain during violent physical effort or severe coughing may be the cause.

Physical Signs.—Pneumo-thorax is a unilateral condition. Inspection shows the intercostal spaces of the affected side obliterated with decided enlargement and immobility. The heart impulse, the liver and spleen are displaced according to the side affected. Palpation, vocal fremitus is diminished or abolished. Percussion over the accumulated air is tympanitic to the line of fluid which yields flatness, varying with the position of the patient. Ausculation reveals absence of vesicular breathing and a faint, distant inspiratory sound of amphoric quality. The rales heard during cough or inspiration are metallic in sound. The metallic tinkle and a splashing sound may be heard by agitating the patient.

The *bruit d'airain* of Trousseau, known as the "coin test," is strongly diagnostic. It consists in tapping one coin against another placed against the chest wall while the ausculator holds an ear over the air-distended area. A clear ringing metallic sound is very conclusive as a diagnostic test.

Symptoms.—If the opening into the pleural cavity is large so that air may pass in and out with each respiration the symptoms may develop slowly, but usually there is a valvular action at the opening so that all the air inspired does not pass out with the subsequent expiration and symptoms of an urgent and alarming nature develop at once, *i. e.*, dyspnœa, pain, faintness, orthopnœa, cyanosis, feeble, rapid pulse, and the patient may die in a few hours from obstructed respiration and collapse. If not so severe, inflammation soon develops with fever, pain, etc., followed by effusion, and the patient dies from pulmonary œdema, cyanosis and the general effects of combined fluid exudate and air pressure.

Prognosis.—This depends upon the history of the case. In healthy individuals there is good hope of recovery if the patient outlives the first few days. The perforation heals, the air is absorbed and the case remains as one of simple pleurisy with effusion or empyema. In cases occurring during the course of phthisis or malignant disease there is but little hope, the patient usually survives only a few days.

Treatment.—The remedies and methods to be employed are the same as in pleurisy with effusion. When the dyspnœa is great, the respiration and pulse rate high and cyanosis and pain are present, the effused air may be aspirated with great relief and good effect.

HÆMO-THORAX.

Definition. — Hæmo-thorax is an accumulation of blood in the pleural cavity.

Etiology.—Due, first, to mechanical injury; second, pulmonary hæmorrhage into the pleural sac, rupture of an aneurism, or erosion of a blood vessel by cancer or tuberculosis. The blood may cause suppuration and rapid death or may be absorbed.

Symptoms.—Are those of hæmorrhage, with symptoms of lung compression and pleuritic effusion added.

Prognosis.—If the hæmorrhage into the pleura is of pulmonary origin, air enters also and the whole situation is most unfavorable; also in aneurism, which is rapidly fatal. From trauma the prognosis is more favorable.

Diagnosis.—This is made on the evidence of rapid effusion after injury, without signs of pleuritis, or in association with intra-thoracic aneurism or malignant disease.

General Treatment.—Consists of absolute rest, ice-bags to the chest, if the diagnosis is sure. Aspiration may be resorted to if necessary.

Remedies.—*Hamamelis*, *Secale*, *Ipecac* or *China* according to their special indications.

V.

Diseases of the Mediastinum.

V.

DISEASES OF THE MEDIASTINUM.

ADENITIS.

The lymphatic glands lying in the mediastinum, along the spine and about the bronchi are involved in all inflammatory diseases of the bronchi and lungs. In broncho-pneumonia and the bronchitis of whooping cough and measles they are particularly prone to become swollen and inflamed, contributing by their presence and pressure to the severity of the cough. In tuberculosis of the lungs they are secondarily involved, becoming the seat of tubercular change, often showing foci of caseous degeneration.

In most cases the simple adenitis of these glands subsides with the primary lesion, with which it is associated. In tuberculosis they may suppurate, the contents being absorbed or undergoing calcification, or, more seriously, perforate into the œsophagus or bronchus.

CARCINOMA OR SARCOMA.

Usually secondary to cancer elsewhere and originating in the thymus gland, lymph glands, pleura or lung. Most frequent in males between the thirtieth and fortieth year.

Symptoms.—The symptoms are those of intra-thoracic pressure:—dyspnœa, cough, aphonia, dysphagia, plus the symptoms of venous obstruction, *i. e.*, cyanosis of the upper part of the body, with distention of the superficial veins.

Diagnosis.—From aneurism is very difficult. If the condition exists over eighteen months it is aneurism. Tumor has not the diastolic shock nor distinct expansile pulsation of aneurism.

ABSCESS.

Abscess may occur and is usually due to trauma. Abscess usually forms in the anterior mediastinum. Pain, throbbing in character, with fever, chills, sweats and dyspnœa. Pus may erode the sternum, perforate an intercostal space or burrow into the abdomen.

EMPHYSEMA.

May occur from trauma, diphtheria, whooping cough, in pneumo-thorax or after tracheotomy.

INDEX.

A.

B.

C.

D.

E.

S.

T.

W.

X.